THE CHILDREN'S HOSPITAL OAKLAND

HEMATOLOGY/ ONCOLOGY HANDBOOK

D1057532

THE CHILDREN'S HOSPITAL OAKLAND

HEMATOLOGY/ ONCOLOGY HANDBOOK

Caroline Hastings, MD

Pediatric Hematologist/Oncologist
Children's Hospital Oakland

Director, Pediatric Hematology and
Oncology Fellowship Program
Children's Hospital Oakland

Member
Children's Oncology Group

Associate Clinical Professor of Pediatrics
University of California, San Francisco
San Francisco, California

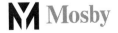 Mosby

An Imprint of Elsevier Science

St. Louis   London   Philadelphia   Sydney   Toronto

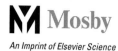

An Imprint of Elsevier Science

Copyright © 2002 by Mosby, Inc.

Mosby, Inc.
An Imprint of Elsevier Science
11830 Westline Industrial Drive
St. Louis, Missouri 63146

Printed in the United States of America

Last digit is the print number: 9   8   7   6   5   4   3   2   1

To my daughters
Leah, Natalie and Juliet
and my husband **Ward**
for your patience, guidance and inspiration.

PREFACE

The pace of change in the field of pediatric hematology and oncology is staggering. Molecular biology, genomics, and biochemistry have accelerated the accumulation of knowledge and understanding of disease states. Yet the application of this new knowledge to the individual child before you, the work of the physician, is often overwhelming, even for the more experienced practitioner. The course and prognosis for the child is often determined by the rapidity of disease onset, diagnosis, and initial treatment. What is needed is a practical, tested approach to these problems that ensures timely evaluation, competent early care, and avoidance of the pitfalls that may prejudice future treatment options. This practical approach is dearly bought by spending time with the patients and their families, and observing the myriad variations that are never mentioned in the large studies or case reports.

This handbook represents the work of my colleagues at Children's Hospital Oakland toward this endeavor. The guidelines offered here have been used to train medical students, pediatric residents, and pediatric hematology and oncology fellows for over 10 years. This handbook will give you clinical approaches to common problems in pediatric hematology and oncology, the knowledge to organize and to evaluate the care of your patients, and a framework to incorporate ever-expanding psychosocial needs, clinical studies, medical treatments, and science. All of these are essential components that make up the care of the child with cancer or blood disease.

Caroline Hastings, MD

CONTENTS

Preface   vii

1   ANEMIA 1

Iron Deficiency Anemia   1
Evaluation   2
Interventions   6

2   HEMOLYTIC ANEMIA 11

Inherited Intracorpuscular Defects   11
Evaluation   14
Treatment   16

3   SICKLE CELL DISEASE 19

Fever and Infection in Sickle Cell Disease   20
Vaso-Occlusive Episodes   22
Acute Chest Syndrome/Pneumonia   26
Priapism   30
Stroke (Cerebrovascular Accident)   30
Acute Anemia   32
Avascular Necrosis   33
Retinopathy/Hyphema   34
Hyperbilirubinemia/Gallstones   35
Perioperative Care for Sickle Cell Patients   35
Transfusion Therapy   36

4   THALASSEMIA 39

α-Thalassemia   39
β-Thalassemia   42
Neonatal Screening for Hemoglobinopathies   45

5   TRANSFUSION THERAPY 47

Blood Products   47
Red Blood Cells   47
Platelets   51
Granulocytes   52
Plasma   53
Antithrombin III   54
Preparation of Blood Products   54

Contents

6   TRANSFUSION REACTIONS **57**

Allergic Reactions   57
Febrile Nonhemolytic Reactions   57
Acute Hemolytic Transfusion Reactions   59
Delayed Transfusion Reactions   59
Alloimmunization   59
Graft-Versus-Host Disease   60
Bacterial Contamination   60

7   CHELATION THERAPY **61**

Chelation for Transfusional Iron Overload   61
Chelation for Acute Lead Toxicity   62

8   THE CHILD WITH A BLEEDING DISORDER **67**

Initial Evaluation   67
Laboratory Evaluation   68

9   von WILLEBRAND DISEASE **75**

Clinical Presentation   75
Diagnosis   76
Treatment   76
Acquired von Willebrand Disease   78

10   HEMOPHILIAS **79**

Hemophilia A and B   79
Hemophilia C (Factor XI Deficiency)   80
Factor XIII Deficiency (Fibrin-Stabilizing Factor)   80
Other Rare Coagulation Abnormalities   81

**11   MANAGEMENT OF ACUTE HEMORRHAGE IN BLEEDING
DIATHESES** **83**

Complications of Bleeding Diatheses   83
Treatment   85
Inhibitors   88
Epistaxis   89

12   THE CHILD WITH THROMBOSIS **93**

Evaluation and Management of the Child with Thrombophilia   93
Guidelines for Anticoagulation Therapy for Venous
   Thromboembolism in Children   95

13 NEUTROPENIA 101

Chronic Benign Neutropenia of Childhood   101
Extrinsic Causes of Neutropenia   102
Diagnostic Approach to the Child with Neutropenia   104
Management of the Child with Neutropenia   104

14 IMMUNE-MEDIATED THROMBOCYTOPENIA......................107

Immune Thrombocytopenic Purpura   107
Chronic Idiopathic Thrombocytopenic Purpura   113
Neonatal Alloimmune Thrombocytopenia   113
Drug-Induced Thrombocytopenia   115

15 NON–IMMUNE-MEDIATED THROMBOCYTOPENIA 117

Increased Platelet Consumption   117
Decreased Platelet Consumption   118

**16 INITIAL EVALUATION OF THE CHILD WITH
     A SUSPECTED MALIGNANCY** 119

Presentation   119
Evaluation of the Child with Suspected Leukemia   122
Evaluation of the Child with an Abdominal Mass   124

17 SUPPORTIVE CARE OF THE CHILD WITH CANCER 127

Infection Prophylaxis   127
Antiemetics   131
Guidelines for Use of Hematopoietic Growth Factors in Children
   with Cancer   135

18 CENTRAL VENOUS CATHETERS 141

Maintenance   141
Complications   141

19 MANAGEMENT OF FEVER IN THE CHILD WITH CANCER ...145

Fever and Neutropenia   145
Fever in the Non-Neutropenic Oncology Patient   151
Prevention of Infection   152

20 ONCOLOGIC EMERGENCIES 153

Superior Vena Cava Syndrome   153
Abdominal Emergencies/Typhlitis   154
Hyperleukocytosis   155
Tumor Lysis Syndrome   157

Contents

21 ACUTE LEUKEMIA 161

Acute Lymphoblastic Leukemia   161
Acute Myelogenous Leukemia   166

22 CENTRAL NERVOUS SYSTEM TUMORS....................171

Clinical Presentation   171
Diagnostic Evaluation   172
Treatment   173
Medulloblastomas   173
Astrocytomas   174
Ependymomas   175

23 HODGKIN'S AND NON-HODGKIN'S LYMPHOMAS..............177

Hodgkin's Disease   177
Non-Hodgkin's Lymphoma   180

24 WILMS' TUMOR 183

Genetics   183
Clinical Presentation   183
Evaluation of Suspected Wilms' Tumor   183
Staging   184
Treatment   185

25 NEUROBLASTOMA 187

Clinical Presentation   187
Diagnostic Evaluation   188
Staging   189
Treatment   189
Prognosis   190

26 GUIDE TO ONCOLOGIC PROCEDURES 191

Intrathecal Chemotherapy   191
Intra-Ommaya Reservoir Tap and Injection
   of Chemotherapy   193
Bone Marrow Aspirate and Biopsy   193
Administration of Peripheral Chemotherapy (in a child without
   a central venous catheter)   195

27 TREATMENT OF CHEMOTHERAPY EXTRAVASATIONS.......197

Formulary Index   199

Formulary   203

Index   257

ANEMIA

Anemia is the condition in which the concentration of hemoglobin or the red cell mass is reduced below normal. Anemia results in a physiologic decrease in the oxygen-carrying capacity of the blood and reduced oxygen supply to the tissues. Causes of anemia are increased loss or destruction of red blood cells (RBCs) or a significantly decreased rate of production. When evaluating a child with anemia, it is important to determine if the problem is isolated to one cell line (e.g., RBCs) or exists in multiple cell lines (i.e., red cells, platelets, white cells). When two or three cell lines are affected, this may indicate bone marrow involvement (i.e., leukemia, metastatic disease, aplastic anemia), sequestration (e.g., hypersplenism), immune deficiency, immune hemolytic anemia, or peripheral destruction of cells (i.e., immune thrombocytopenic purpura).

IRON DEFICIENCY ANEMIA

Iron deficiency is the most common form of anemia and exceeds all other causes in childhood by a factor of at least three. As the amount of iron in the newborn is approximately 75 mg/kg, a 3-kg infant will have approximately 225 mg total body iron at birth. If there is no iron in the diet, or if iron loss is greater than iron intake, by 6 months in full-term infants and as early as 3–4 months in premature infants, the iron stores present at birth will be depleted. The most common cause of iron deficiency is inadequate intake of iron during the rapidly growing childhood years. Excessive consumption of cow's milk associated with gastroenteritis and chronic blood loss and blood loss due to underlying diseases through the gastrointestinal tract, lungs, or kidney should be considered.

Iron reserves begin to decrease during the early stages of iron deficiency, resulting in a low serum ferritin concentration. Values less than 12 mg/mL have been considered diagnostic of iron deficiency. However, normal ferritin levels can exist in iron-deficient states when coexisting with a bacterial or parasitic infection, malignancy, or chronic inflammatory condition, as ferritin is an acute-phase reactant. As serum iron concentrations decrease, transferrin (total iron binding capacity [TIBC]) synthesis is stimulated, and the iron-transferrin ratio, called the transferrin saturation, decreases. A transferrin saturation less than 10% is consistent with iron deficiency.

The FEP concentration increases when the iron supply is low enough to impede Hb synthesis. The FEP is a simple, sensitive test for iron deficiency and can provide a guide to the adequacy of iron replacement therapy.

With pronounced iron deficiency, the peripheral blood smear is remarkable for a microcytic, hypochromic anemia with severe anisocytosis and poikilocytosis. Basophilic stippling can occur, making such cases quite similar to thalassemia trait. Iron deficiency occurs over time; therefore, the red cell size is varied and the RDW is very high (>14). This is in contrast to the thalassemia traits, in which the RDW is normal.

Physical findings associated wtih iron deficiency include pallor, lethargy, tachycardia, and tachypnea. Because iron deficiency develops over time, cardiorespiratory compensation is often quite remarkable, and some patients can tolerate Hb concentrations as low as 4 g/dL. In some cases of iron deficiency, growth retardation and neurodevelopmental delay can occur. In addition, protein-losing enteropathy can result as a consequence of iron depletion in the cells lining the gastrointestinal tract. Iron stores will be depleted before development of anemia, placing the infant at risk for the nonhematologic effects of iron deficiency.

EVALUATION

The evaluation of anemia includes a complete medical history, family history, physical examination, and laboratory assessment (Fig. 1–1).

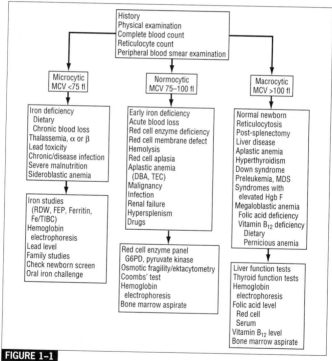

FIGURE 1–1

Diagnostic approach to the child with anemia. (Abbreviations: MCV = mean cell volume; DBA = Diamond-Blackfan anemia; TEC = transient erythroblastopenia of childhood; MDS, myelodysplastic syndrome; Hgb F = hemoglobin F; RDW = red cell distribution index; FEP = free erythrocyte protoporphyrin; Fe/TIBC = iron-/total iron-binding capacity; G6PD = glucose-6-phosphate dehydrogenase.)

TABLE 1-1

NORMAL RED BLOOD CELL VALUES IN CHILDREN

AGE	HEMOGLOBIN (g/dl)		MCV (fl)	
	Mean	−2 SD	Mean	−2 SD
Birth (cord blood)	16.5	13.5	108	98
1–3 days (capillary)	18.5	14.5	108	95
1 week	17.5	13.5	107	88
2 weeks	16.5	12.5	105	86
1 month	14.0	10.0	104	85
2 months	11.5	9.0	96	77
3–6 months	11.5	9.5	91	74
0.5–2 years	12.0	10.5	78	70
2–6 years	12.5	11.5	81	75
6–12 years	13.5	11.5	86	77
12–18 years, female	14.0	12.0	90	78
12–18 years, male	14.5	13.0	88	78
18–49 years, female	14.0	12.0	90	80
18–49 years, male	15.5	13.5	90	80

Compiled from several sources; the mean ± 2 SD can be expected to include 95% of the observations in a normal population. Adapted from Hastings CA, Lubin BH. Blood. In: Rudolph AM, Kamei RK (eds), Rudolph's Fundamentals of Pediatrics, 2nd ed. Norwalk, CT: Appleton & Lange, 1998, pp 441–490.
MCV = mean corpuscular volume.

1

EVALUATION

The diagnosis of anemia is made after reference to established normal RBC control values for age (Table 1–1). The blood smear and red cell indices are very helpful in the diagnosis and classification of anemia. They allow for classification by cell size (mean cell volume [MCV]) and may give important diagnostic clues if specific morphologic abnormalities are present (e.g., sickle cells, target cells, spherocytes). The MCV and reticulocyte count are helpful in the differential diagnosis of anemia. A normal or low reticulocyte count is an inappropriate response to anemia and suggests impaired red cell production. An elevated reticulocyte count suggests blood loss, hemolysis, or sequestration.

The investigation of anemia requires the following steps:

1. The medical history of the anemic child (Table 1–2); certain historical points may provide clues as to the etiology of the anemia.
2. Detailed physical examination (Table 1–3), with particular attention to acute and chronic effects of anemia.
3. Evaluation of the complete blood count (CBC), RBC indices, and peripheral blood smear, with classification by MCV, reticulocyte count, and RBC morphology. Consideration should also be given to the white cell and platelet counts and morphology.

TABLE 1–2

THE MEDICAL HISTORY OF THE ANEMIC CHILD

HISTORY OF	CONSIDER
Prematurity	Anemia of prematurity (EPO responsive)
Perinatal risk factors	
Maternal illness (autoimmune)	Hemolytic anemia
Drug ingestion	Impaired production
Infections (TORCH, rubella, CMV, hepatitis)	
Perinatal problems	Acute blood loss
	Fetal–maternal hemorrhage
	Iron deficiency caused by above or maternal iron deficiency
Ethnicity	
American black	Hgb S, C; α, β thal; G6PD deficiency
Mediterranean	α, β thal; G6PD deficiency
Southeast Asian	α, β thal; Hgb E
Family history	
Gallstones, cholecystectomy	Inherited hemolytic anemia, spherocytosis, elliptocytosis
Splenectomy, jaundice at birth or with illness	Inherited enzymopathy: G6PD, pyruvate kinase deficiencies; inherited red cell membrane defect: spherocytosis, elliptocytosis
Isoimmunization (Rh or ABO)	Hemolytic disease of newborn (Predisposed to iron deficiency)
Sex	
Male	X-linked enzymopathies (G6PD)
Early jaundice (<24 hours of age)	Isoimmune, infectious
Persistent jaundice	Hemolytic anemia
Diet (usually >6 months)	
Pica (ice, dirt)	Lead toxicity, iron deficiency
Excessive milk intake	Iron deficiency
Macrobiotic diets	Vitamin B_{12} deficiency
Goat's milk	Folic acid deficiency
Drugs	
Sulfa, anticonvulsants	Hemolytic anemia (G6PD)
Chloramphenicol	Hypoplastic anemia
Low socioeconomic status	
Pica	Lead toxicity, iron deficiency
Malnutrition	
Malabsorption	Anemia of chronic disease
Environmental	Iron, B_{12}, or folate deficiency, vitamin E or K deficiency
Liver disease	Shortened red cell survival, Heinz bodies
Renal disease	Shortened red cell survival
Decreased red cell production ($\downarrow$ EPO)	

Table continued on opposite page

TABLE 1–2
THE MEDICAL HISTORY OF THE ANEMIC CHILD Continued

HISTORY OF	CONSIDER
Infectious diseases	
Mild viral infection (acute gastroenteritis, otitis media, pharyngitis)	Transient mild decreased Hgb
Sepsis (bacterial, viral, mycoplasma)	Hemolytic anemia
Parvovirus	Anemia with reticulocytopenia (TEC)

Abbreviations: EPO = erythropoietin; TORCH = toxoplasmosis, other viruses, rubella, cytomegalovirus, and herpes simplex; CMV, cytomegalovirus; Hgb = hemoglobin; thal = thalassemia; G6PD = glucose-6-phosphate dehydrogenase; TEC = transient erythroblastopenia of childhood.
Adapted from Hastings CA, Lubin BH. Blood. In: Rudolph AM, Kamei RK (eds), Rudolph's Fundamentals of Pediatrics, 2nd ed. Norwalk, CT: Appleton & Lange, 1998, pp 441–490.

TABLE 1–3
PHYSICAL EXAMINATION OF THE ANEMIC CHILD

	PHYSICAL FINDING	CONSIDER
Skin	Pallor	Severe anemia
	Jaundice	Hemolytic anemia, acute & chronic Hepatitis, aplastic anemia
	Petechiae, purpura	Autoimmune hemolytic anemia with thrombocytopenia
		Hemolytic–uremic syndrome
		Bone marrow aplasia or infiltration
	Cavernous hemangioma	Microangiopathic hemolytic anemia
HEENT	Frontal bossing, prominent malar and maxillary bones	Extramedullary hematopoiesis (thalassemia major, congenital hemolytic anemia)
	Icteric sclerae	Congenital hemolytic anemia and/or hyperhemolytic crises associated with infection (red cell enzyme deficiencies, red cell membrane defects, thalassemias, hemoglobinopathies)
	Angular stomatitis	Iron deficiency
	Glossitis	Vitamin B_{12} or iron deficiency
Chest	Rales, gallop rhythm	Congestive heart failure, acute or severe anemia
	Tachycardia	
Extremities	Radial limb dysplasia	Fanconi's anemia
	Spoon nails	Iron deficiency
	Triphalangeal thumbs	Red cell aplasia
Spleen	Splenomegaly	Congenital hemolytic anemia, infection, hematologic malignancies, portal hypertension with resultant hypersplenism

Adapted from Hastings CA, Lubin BH. Blood. In: Rudolph AM, Kamei RK (eds), Rudolph's Fundamentals of Pediatrics, 2nd ed. Norwalk, CT: Appleton & Lange, 1998, pp 441–490.

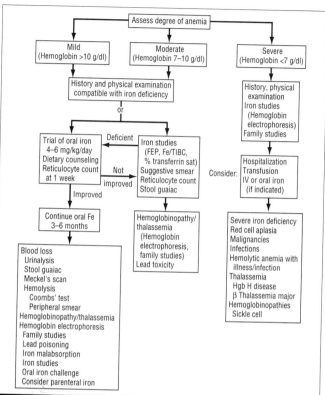

FIGURE 1–2

Diagnostic approach to the child with microcytic anemia. (Abbreviations: FEP = free erthyrocyte protoporphyrin; Fe/TIBC = iron-/total iron-binding capacity; Hgb H = hemoglobin H.)

4. Determination of etiology of the anemia by additional studies as needed (Figs. 1–2 and 1–3).

INTERVENTIONS

ORAL IRON THERAPY

Treatment of iron deficiency requires identification and correction of nutritional inadequacies, search for blood loss, and therapy with iron (2 mg elemental iron/kg twice daily). Iron therapy should be continued for several months after the red cell indices return to normal. Failure to respond to iron often reflects poor compliance. However, it may mean that the response is blunted by infection or that the diagnosis is incorrect. An adequate response to iron therapy is reflected by an increase of Hb concentration greater than 1 g/dL in 10 days. If measured, a reticulocytosis is usually evident within 3–5 days after starting oral iron supplementation. The FEP returns to normal when iron deficiency is corrected.

ORAL IRON CHALLENGE

An oral iron challenge may be indicated in the patient with significant iron depletion, as documented by moderate to severe anemia and deficiencies in circulating and storage iron forms (total iron-binding capacity, serum iron, transferrin saturation, ferritin). Iron absorption is impaired in certain chronic disorders (peptic ulcer disease, ulcerative colitis, Crohn's disease), by certain medications (antacids, histamine-2 blockers), and by environmental factors such as lead toxicity.

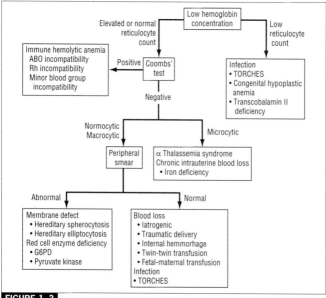

FIGURE 1–3

Diagnostic approach to the full-term newborn with anemia. (Abbreviations: TORCHES = toxoplasmosis, other viruses, rubella, cytomegalovirus, herpes simplex virus; G6PD = glucose-6-phosphate dehydrogenase.)

Indications
Indications for an oral iron challenge include any condition in which a poor response to oral iron is being questioned, such as

1. Noncompliance
2. Severe anemia secondary to dietary insufficiency (excessive milk intake)
3. Ongoing blood loss

To administer an oral iron challenge is quite simple. First, draw a serum iron level, then administer a dose of iron (4 to 6 mg/kg elemental iron) orally, and then draw another serum iron level 30 to 60 minutes later. The serum level is expected to increase by at least 100 μg/dl if absorption is adequate. The oral iron challenge is a quick and easy method to assess appropriateness of oral iron to treat iron deficiency—a safer and cheaper method of treatment than parenteral iron, yet equally efficacious.

PARENTERAL IRON THERAPY
Iron dextran, a parenteral form of elemental iron, is available for IM or IV administration. The preferred route is IV because of the painful nature of the injection and longstanding skin discoloration. A simple formula for dosage is

$$\text{Dose of iron (mg)} = \text{weight (kg)} \times \text{desired increment hemoglobin (g/dl)} \times 2.5$$

Add 10 mg/kg to replenish iron stores (chronic anemia states). The maximum adult dose is 14 ml. Each milliliter of iron dextran contains 50 mg elemental iron. Replacement may be able to be given in a single dose, depending on the dose required (see Formulary for more dosing information). A dosing chart is also available in the *Physicians' Desk Reference*.

Peak reticulocytosis occurs after 10 days, and complete correction of the anemia may be seen in 3 to 4 weeks. The hemoglobin may be increased in 1 to 2 weeks.

Severe allergic reactions can occur with iron dextran. A test dose (12.5 to 25 mg) is frequently given, with observation of the patient for 30 to 60 minutes prior to administering the remainder of the dose. A common side effect is mild to moderate arthralgias the day after drug administration, especially in patients with autoimmune disease. Acetaminophen frequently alleviates the arthralgias. Iron dextran is contraindicated in patients with rheumatoid arthritis.

ERYTHROPOIETIN
Recombinant human erythropoietin (EPO) stimulates proliferation and differentiation of erythroid precursors, with an increase in heme synthesis. This increased proliferation creates an increased demand for iron availability and

can result in a functional iron deficiency if EPO is not given with iron therapy.

Indications for EPO include

1. End-stage renal disease
2. Anemia of prematurity
3. Anemia of chronic disease
4. Anemia associated with treatment for acquired immunodeficiency syndrome
5. Sickle cell disease/thalassemia
6. Autologous blood donation

EPO is currently under investigation for the treatment of chemotherapy-induced anemia.

The most common side effect of EPO administration is hypertension, which may be somewhat alleviated with changes in the dose and duration of administration.

A typical starting dose of EPO is 150 U/kg three times a week IV or SQ. CBCs and reticulocyte counts are checked weekly. Higher doses, and more frequent dosing, may be necessary. Response is usually seen within 1 to 2 weeks. Adequate iron intake (3 mg/kg/day orally or intermittent parenteral therapy) should be provided to optimize effectiveness and prevent iron deficiency.

TRANSFUSION THERAPY

Children with very severe anemia (hemoglobin <5 g/dl) may require treatment with red cell transfusion, depending on the underlying disease and baseline hemoglobin status, duration of anemia, rapidity of onset, and hemodynamic stability. The pediatric literature is scarce as to the best method of transfusing such patients. However, it appears to be common practice to give slow transfusions to children with cardiovascular compromise (gallop, pulmonary edema, excessive tachycardia, poor perfusion) while they are being monitored in an intensive care unit setting. Transfusions are given in multiple small volumes, sometimes separated by several hours, with careful monitoring of the vital signs and fluid balance. For those children who have gradual onset of severe anemia without cardiovascular compromise, continuous transfusion of 2 ml/kg/hour has been shown to be safe and to result in an increase in the hematocrit of 1% for each 1 ml/kg of transfused packed RBCs. The hemoglobin should be increased to a normal value (8 to 12 g/dl) to avoid further cardiac compromise. Again, the final endpoint may be dependent on several factors, including nature of anemia, ongoing blood loss or lack of production, baseline hemoglobin, and volume to be transfused. Care should be taken to avoid unnecessary exposure to multiple blood donors by maximal use of the unit of blood, proper division of units in the blood bank, and avoidance of opening extra units for small quantities to meet a total volume. (See Chapter 5 for product preparation, ordering, and premedication.) A hemoglobin should be checked 2 to 4 hours after completion of the transfusion to allow for equilibration and assure an appropriate rise.

SUGGESTED READING

Hastings CA, Lubin BH. Blood. In: Rudolph AM, Kamei RK (eds), Rudolph's Fundamentals of Pediatrics, 2nd ed. Norwalk, CT: Appleton & Lange, 1998, pp 441–490.

Jayabose S, Tugal O, Ruddy R, et al. Transfusion therapy for severe anemia. Am J Pediatr Hematol Oncol 15:324–327, 1993.

Lanzkowsky P. Manual of Pediatric Hematology and Oncology, 3rd ed. San Diego: Academic Press, 2000.

Oski FA, Brugnara C, Nathan DG. A diagnostic approach to the anemic patient. In: Nathan DG, Orkin SH (eds), Nathan and Oski's Hematology of Infancy and Childhood, 5th ed. Philadelphia: WB Saunders, 1998, pp 373–496.

HEMOLYTIC ANEMIA

Red blood cells normally live 100 to 120 days in the circulation. Hemolytic anemia results from a reduced red cell survival or increased destruction. To compensate, the bone marrow increases its output of red cells, a response mediated by erythropoietin. Destruction of red cells occurs intravascularly (within the circulation) or extravascularly (by phagocytic cells of the bone marrow, liver, or spleen). Red cell injury or destruction is associated with transformation to a rigid or abnormal form. Altered cell deformability then leads to decreased survival. Hemolytic anemia may be inherited (thalassemias, hemoglobinopathies, red cell enzyme deficiencies, membrane defects), or acquired (immune mediated, associated with infection or medications). It can be chronic or acute. Some types of low-grade chronic hemolytic anemias can have acute exacerbations, such as in a child with glucose-6-phosphate dehydrogenase (G6PD) deficiency following an exposure to fava beans or naphthalene.

INHERITED INTRACORPUSCULAR DEFECTS

RED CELL MEMBRANE DISORDERS

Hereditary spherocytosis (HS) is the most common congenital red blood cell membrane disorder. Another membrane defect, hereditary elliptocytosis (HE), is seen infrequently and characterized by classical elliptocytic red cells in the peripheral blood smear with reticulocytosis and a clinical variability of expression of the hemolytic anemia. The usual patient with HS has intermittent jaundice, as well as hemolytic and/or red cell aplastic episodes associated with viral infection, splenomegaly, and cholelithiasis. However, the clinical presentation is quite variable, with most severe cases presenting in the newborn period or early childhood and milder cases presenting in adulthood.

Several membrane protein defects are responsible for HS. Most result in instability of spectrin, one of the major skeletal membrane proteins. Structural changes that result as a consequence of protein deficiency lead to membrane instability, loss of surface area, abnormal membrane permeability, and decreased red cell deformability. Metabolic depletion accentuates the defect in HS cells, which accounts for an increase in osmotic fragility after a 24-hour incubation of whole blood at 37°C. The splenic sinusoids prevent passage of nondeformable spherocytic red cells. This explains the occurrence of splenomegaly in HS and the therapeutic effect of splenectomy.

Patients with HS have a mild to moderate chronic hemolytic anemia. Red cell indices reveal a decreased mean cell volume (MCV). Cellular dehydration increases the mean cellular concentration of hemoglobin, characteristically by more than 36%. The red cell distribution width is elevated because of the variable presence of microspheres in proportion to the degree of hemolysis. A recently developed test performed on an ektacytometer measures the deformity of red cells subjected simultaneously to shear stress and osmotic stress. Osmotic fragility tests and ektactyometry studies are characteristic for HS, with increased fragility in hypotonic environments.

As with other hemolytic anemias, affected individuals are susceptible to hypoplastic crises during viral infections. Human parvovirus B19, a frequent pathogen and the organism responsible for erythema infectiosum, selectively invades erythroid progenitor cells and may result in a transient arrest in red cell proliferation. Recovery begins within 7 to 10 days after infection and is usually complete within 4 to 6 weeks. If the initial presentation of a patient with HS is during an aplastic crisis, a diagnosis of HS might not be considered because the reticulocyte count will be low and the peripheral blood smear may be nondiagnostic. The family history of HS should be explored; if it is suggestive, the patient should be evaluated for HS after recovery from the aplastic episode.

Patients with HS should be counseled regarding signs and symptoms of hemolysis as well as certain precipitating events, and should receive folic acid supplementation (1 mg/day). Splenectomy is often considered for patients who have had severe hemolysis requiring transfusions or repeated hospitalization, or show signs of hypersplenism (thrombocytopenia, leukopenia). In patients with mild hemolysis, the decision to perform splenectomy should be delayed; in many cases splenectomy may not be required. For pediatric patients who have excessive splenic size, an additional consideration for splenectomy is to diminish the risk of traumatic splenic rupture. The risk of splenectomy must be considered before any clinical decision is made regarding the procedure.

Red cell survival returns to normal values after splenectomy unless an accessory spleen develops. Although an increased number of spherocytes can be seen in the peripheral blood after splenectomy and the osmotic fragility is worse, the hemoglobin value is normal. Platelet counts frequently increase to more than 1000×10^9/L immediately after splenectomy but return to normal levels over several weeks. No therapeutic interventions are required for postsplenectomy thrombocytosis in patients with HS.

To minimize the risk of sepsis resulting from *Haemophilus influenzae* and *Streptococcus pneumoniae*, the splenectomy procedure (when necessary) is often postponed until after the child's fifth or sixth birthday. Patients should be immunized against these organisms prior to splenectomy and receive penicillin prophylaxis following the procedure. The increase in penicillin-resistant strains of *S. pneumoniae* has raised questions regarding the use of prophylactic penicillin. No studies have determined the frequency of this problem in children receiving prophylactic penicillin after splenectomy.

RED CELL ENZYME DEFECTS

Glucose is the primary metabolic substrate for the red cell. Because the mature red cell does not contain mitochondria, it can metabolize glucose only by anaerobic mechanisms. The two major metabolic pathways within the red cell are the Embden-Meyerhoff pathway (EMP) and the hexose monophosphate shunt.

Red cell morphologic changes are minimal in patients with red cell enzyme deficiency involving the EMP. Red cell indices are usually normocytic and normochromic. The reticulocyte count is elevated in proportion to the extent of hemolysis. Because many enzyme activities are normally increased in young red cells, a mild deficiency in one of the enzymes may be obscured by the reticulocytosis.

Pyruvate Kinase Deficiency

Pyruvate kinase (PK) deficiency is the most common enzyme deficiency in the EMP. The inheritance pattern of this disorder is autosomal recessive. Homozygotes usually have hemolytic anemia with splenomegaly, whereas the heterozygotes are usually asymptomatic. The disorder is found worldwide, although it is most common in whites of northern European descent. The range of clinical expression is variable, from severe neonatal jaundice to a fully compensated hemolytic anemia. Anemia is usually normochromic and normocytic, but macrocytes may be present shortly after a hemolytic crisis, reflecting erythroid hyperplasia and early release of red cells. The osmotic fragility of red cells is normal or slightly reduced. Diagnosis is confirmed by a quantitative assay for PK.

Splenectomy is a therapeutic option for PK-deficient patients. As with HS, the decision should be made on the basis of the patient's clinical course. Unlike HS patients, PK-deficient patients, although they improve after splenectomy, do not have complete correction of their hemolytic anemia. As with all hemolytic anemias, these patients should have dietary supplementation with folic acid (1 mg/day) to prevent megaloblastic complications associated with relative folate deficiency. Immunization against *H. influenzae* and *S. pneumoniae* should be given, as well as lifelong penicillin prophylaxis in the splenectomized patient.

Glucose-6-Phosphate Dehydrogenase Deficiency

G6PD deficiency, the most common red cell enzyme deficiency, is sex linked, with partial expression in the female population and full expression in the affected male population. The distribution of G6PD deficiency is worldwide, with the highest incidence in Africans and African-Americans. Mediterraneans, American Indians, Southeast Asians, and Sephardic Jews are also affected. In African-Americans, 12% of the male population have the deficiency, 18% of the female population are heterozygotes, and 2% of the female population are homozygous. In Southeast Asians, G6PD deficiency is found in approximately 6% of the male population. One hypothesis for the prevalence of this enzyme abnormality is that it confers resistance to malaria.

Many variants of G6PD deficiency are known and have been characterized at the biochemical and molecular levels. A variant found in Mediterraneans is associated with chronic hemolytic anemia. Other variants are associated with an unstable enzyme that has normal levels in the young red cells. These result in hemolysis only in association with an oxidant chal-

2

INHERITED INTRACORPUSCULAR DEFECTS

lenge (as found in African-Americans). In some cases of G6PD deficiency, hemolysis may be triggered by the oxidant intermediates generated during viral or bacterial infections or after ingestion of oxidant compounds. Shortly after exposure to the oxidant, hemoglobin is oxidized to methemoglobin and eventually denatured, forming intracellular inclusions called Heinz bodies, which attach to the red cell membrane. This portion of the membrane may be removed by the reticuloendothelial cells, resulting in a "bite" cell, which has a shortened survival because of its loss of membrane components. To compensate for hemolysis, red cell production is increased and the reticulocyte count is increased.

Individuals with the Mediterranean or Asian forms of G6PD deficiency, in addition to being sensitive to infections and certain drugs, often have a chronic, moderately severe anemia with nonspherocytic red cells and jaundice. Hemolysis usually starts in early childhood. Reticulocytosis is present and can result in an increase in the MCV.

When a hemolytic crisis occurs in G6PD deficiency or favism, pallor, scleral icterus, hemoglobinemia, hemoglobinuria, and splenomegaly may be noted. Plasma haptoglobin and hemopexin concentrations are low. The peripheral smear shows the fragmented bite cells and polychromatophilic cells. Red cell indices may be normal. Special stains can detect Heinz bodies in the cells during the first few days of hemolysis.

A diagnosis of G6PD deficiency should be based on family history, ethnicity, laboratory features, physical findings, and clinical suspicion following a possible recent exposure to oxidants with resultant acute hemolysis. The diagnosis is confirmed by a quantitative enzyme assay. Treatment is directed toward supportive care for the acute event and counseling regarding prevention of future hemolytic crises. In patients with chronic hemolysis, dietary supplementation with folic acid (1 mg/day) is recommended. Use of vitamin E, 500 mg/day, may improve red cell survival in patients with chronic hemolysis.

EVALUATION

The evaluation of hemolytic anemia includes a thorough history assessing for evidence of chronic hemolytic anemia and possible precipitants of an acute event (Fig. 2–1). The family history is equally important. Questions to ask include those regarding

- History of newborn jaundice
- Gallstones
- Splenomegaly or splenectomy
- Episodes of dark urine and or yellow skin/sclerae
- Anemia unresponsive to iron supplementation
- Medications
- Environmental exposures
- Ethnicity
- Dietary history

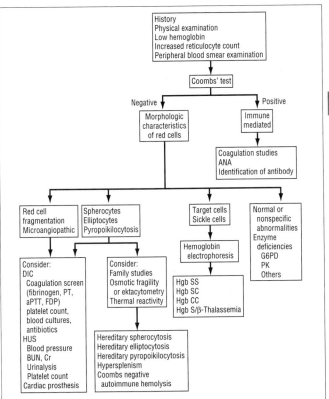

BUN=blood urea nitrogen; Cr=creatinine; EMP=Embden-Meyerhof pathway; FDP=fibrin degradation products; G6PD=glucose—6-phosphate dehydrogenase; Hgb=hemoglobin; HK=hexokinase; HMS hexose monophosphate shunt; PK=pyruvinate kinase; PT=prothrombin time; aPTT=partial prothrombin time. HUS=hemolytic uremic syndrome

FIGURE 2–1

Diagnostic approach to the child with hemolytic anemia. (Abbreviations: ANA = antinuclear antibodies; DIC = disseminated intravascular coagulation; PT = prothrombin time; aPTT = activated partial thromboplastin time; FDP = fibrin degradation product; G6PD = glucose-6-phosphate dehydrogenase; PK = pyruvate kinase; HUS = hemolytic–uremic syndrome; BUN = blood urea nitrogen; Cr = creatinine; Hgb = hemoglobin.) (Adapted from Hastings CA, Lubin BH. Blood. In: Rudolph AM, Kamei RK (eds), Rudolph's Fundamentals of Pediatrics, 2nd ed. Norwalk, CT: Appleton & Lange, 1998, pp 441–490; reprinted with permission.)

The physical exam should be complete, but should be focused on

- Skin color (pallor, jaundice, icteric sclerae)
- Facial bone changes (extramedullary hematopoiesis)
- Abdominal fullness, splenomegaly

The laboratory evaluation includes

- Complete blood count, red cell indices, reticulocyte count (elevated)
- Peripheral blood smear (assess for fragmented forms or evidence of inherited anemia with specific morphologic abnormalities)
- Bilirubin (elevated)
- Coombs' test, direct and indirect (to exclude antibody-mediated red cell destruction)
- Urinalysis (for heme, bilirubin)
- Free plasma hemoglobin (elevated)
- Thermal reactivity to determine warm-reactive (usually IgG) or cold-reactive autoantibodies (IgG or IgM)

Specific tests for diagnosis may include

- Osmotic fragility (HS, HE)
- Ektacytometry (HS, HE)
- Red cell enzyme levels (G6PD, PK)

The osmotic fragility test is used to measure the osmotic resistance of red cells. Red cells are incubated under hypotonic conditions, and their ability to swell before lysis is determined. The osmotic fragility of red cells is increased when the surface area:volume ratio of the red cells is decreased, as in hereditary spherocytosis, in which membrane instability results in membrane loss and decreased surface area. Conversely, osmotic fragility is decreased in liver disease and the ratio of the red cell surface area to volume is increased.

TREATMENT

Therapy is dependent on the underlying nature of the anemia and degree of acute hemolysis. In chronic hemolysis, such as that associated with HS, splenectomy is often recommended to decrease the degree of splenic destruction and degree of anemia, as well as the incidence of bilirubin stones. In other forms of inherited anemias in which the hemolysis is more significant and even life threatening, such as thalassemia or some forms of enzymopathies, chronic transfusion therapy is recommended.

Other general measures include folic acid replacement because of high cell turnover, avoidance of oxidant chemicals and drugs, splenectomy in some cases, and iron chelation therapy as indicated for transfusion-related iron overload.

Immune hemolytic anemias may require more immediate and aggressive therapy. The underlying disease, if present and identifiable, warrants treatment. Additionally, the use of corticosteroids in high doses is frequently necessary. Splenectomy and immunosuppressive drugs have also been successful.

Microangiopathic hemolytic anemias, such as those associated with the hemolytic—remic syndrome, disseminated intravascular coagulopathy, burns, or surgical procedures, can also be severe and life threatening. Striking morphologic abnormalities of the red cells are seen with evidence of intravascular hemolysis (elevated bilirubin, free plasma hemoglobin). Treatment should first be directed toward the primary disorder to remove the cause of the trauma if possible. Transfusions are frequently necessary, and splenectomy may be needed in some patients with severe hypersplenism.

SUGGESTED READING

Hastings CA, Lubin BH. Blood. In: Rudolph AM, Kamei RK (eds), Rudolph's Fundamentals of Pediatrics, 2nd ed. Norwalk, CT: Appleton & Lange, 1998, pp 441–490.

Oski FA, Brugnara C, Nathan DG. A diagnostic approach to the anemic patient. In: Nathan DG, Orkin SH (eds), Nathan and Oski's Hematology of Infancy and Childhood, 5th ed. Philadelphia: WB Saunders, 1998, pp 373–496.

SICKLE CELL DISEASE

Sickle cell disease refers to a group of genetic disorders that share a common feature: hemoglobin S (Hgb S), alone or in combination with another abnormal hemoglobin. The sickle cell diseases are inherited in an autosomal codominant manner. The molecular defect in Hgb S is due to the substitution of valine for glutamic acid in the sixth position of the β-globin chain. This substitution results in polymerization of the hemoglobin and causes the red cells to transform from deformable biconcave disks into rigid, sickle-shaped cells. Hypoxia, acidosis, and hypertonicity facilitate polymer formation.

The most common combinations of hemoglobins are: (1) Hgb SS, (2) Hgb SC, and (3) Hgb S with a β-thalassemia, either $S\beta^+$ or $S\beta^0$. The most severely affected individuals have either Hgb SS or $S\beta^0$ (no normal β-globin production). Individuals with Hgb $S\beta^+$ have decreased β-globin production and less severe disease, whereas children who have Hgb SC have intermediate severity of their disease. There is overlap between Hgb SS and Hgb SC; some children who have Hgb SC are more symptomatic than children who have Hgb SS. There are many **variables to expression** of this hemoglobinopathy, including haplotypes, Hgb F concentration, and other yet-to-be-defined factors. It is not possible to predict the severity of disease in advance of severe complications. Generally, children who have vaso-occlusion and other complications have a more severe course. Increased leukocyte count and frequency and severity of vaso-occlusive episodes (VOEs) are associated with increased morbidity and mortality.

α-Thalassemia (frequency 1% to 3% in African-Americans) may be co-inherited with sickle cell trait or disease. Individuals who have both α-thalassemia and sickle cell anemia are less anemic that those who have sickle cell anemia alone. However, α-thalassemia trait does not appear to prevent frequency or severity of vaso-occlusive complications of organ damage.

Sickle cell disease is not uncommon. In African-Americans, the frequency of the sickle cell gene is 8%; that of the Hgb C gene, 4%; and that of the β-thalassemia gene, 1%. Approximately 1 in 600 African-American infants has sickle cell anemia. Sickle cell disease also occurs in children from the Middle East, India, Central and South America, and the Caribbean.

All children who have sickle cell hemoglobinopathies have a variable degree of hemolytic anemia and vaso-occlusive tissue ischemia resulting in the numerous clinical complications. Organs most sensitive to the ischemic–hypoxic injury of red cell sickling are the lungs, spleen, kidney, bone marrow, eyes, brain, and heads of the humerus and femur. Sickling has both acute and long-term implications for organ function. **Cerebral vascular disease** can be subtle, causing only abnormal neuropsychological testing, or it can be catastrophic, resulting in hemiparesis, coma, or

3

death. Acute **pulmonary sickling** causes lung injury eventually leading to pulmonary hypertension. **Osteonecrosis** of the femoral head can be debilitating, leading to the need for hip replacement. Untreated **retinopathy** can lead to blindness, and sickle cell **nephropathy** can eventually lead to renal failure.

Now that newborn hemoglobinopathy testing is mandatory in most states, children are diagnosed early and receive appropriate care before they are at risk for complications. All infants who have an electrophoretic pattern of Hgb FS at birth will have some form of sickle cell disease.

Baseline hemoglobin values for children with sickle cell disease are dependent on the coexistence of Hgb C or thalassemia. The following are relative steady-state values, though individuals should be monitored periodically to establish their own baseline normal values, which are helpful for comparison in the ill state.

Genotype	Average Hgb (g/dl)	Reticulocyte Count (%)
Hgb SS	8–10	10–25
Hgb SC	10–12	5–10
Hgb Sβ^0	8–10	10–15
Hgb Sβ$^+$	10–12	3–6
Hgb SS/α-thalassemia	8–9	5–10

FEVER AND INFECTION IN SICKLE CELL DISEASE

Susceptibility to infection is increased primarily because of splenic infarction, but also because of other acquired immunologic abnormalities. This can result in life-threatening episodes of sepsis. Recognition of this susceptibility and aggressive medical management have resulted in an increased life span for most patients.

Most children with sickle cell disease are identified at birth, started on prophylactic penicillin by age 2 months, and aggressively monitored and treated for signs of infection. However, with the increasing problems of bacterial antibiotic resistance, health care providers need to be vigilant when confronted with an infant or child who has a fever (38.5°C orally) or appears ill. Overall, *Streptococcus pneumoniae* is responsible for more than 80% of the morbidity of infection. In some areas of the country, up to 50% of pneumococcal isolates are penicillin resistant. Infections can precipitate VOEs and other complications of sickle cell anemia and, in this population, can quickly become fulminant.

Bacteria that cause the most morbidity and mortality include *S. pneumoniae, Haemophilus influenzae, Neisseria meningitidis, Mycoplasma pneumoniae, Staphylococcus aureus, Salmonella* species, *Escherichia coli,* and *Streptococcus pyogenes.* The *H. influenzae* type B vaccine has resulted in a lowered case rate of sepsis from this organism, and it is anticipated that the new polysaccharide pneumococcal vaccine will have a similar positive outcome. Viral infections, particularly parvovirus B19, can cause severe aplastic crises as well as acute chest syndrome (ACS).

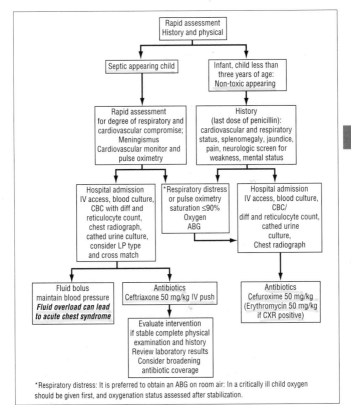

FIGURE 3–1

Approach to fever in a child with sickle cell disease. (Abbreviations: CBC = complete blood count; diff = differential; LP = lumbar puncture; ABG = arterial blood gas; CXR = chest x-ray.)

Infants, young children, and any patient who has a central venous catheter who present with a fever (≥38.5°C orally) should have a complete evaluation. Laboratory studies should include complete blood count (CBC) with differential, reticulocyte count, blood culture, urinalysis, and urine culture (Fig. 3–1). A chest radiograph should also be obtained. Meningitis occurs in children who have sickle cell disease, but routine lumbar punctures without physical signs of meningitis are not warranted. Urosepsis is common in sickle cell patients of all ages. All infants should be admitted, started on parenteral antibiotics, have cultures followed for 48 to 72 hours, and not be discharged during this time even if they appear well and are afebrile.

Children who have a fever should have the same work-up as infants. ACS should be high on the differential in all children who have a fever. Although physical examination is essential, 60% of pulmonary infiltrates in children with sickle cell disease and fever will be missed on exam alone. If there is another possible source of infection, appropriate cultures should be obtained. If a child appears to be ill, has an oral temperature of 38.5°C or higher, or has an elevated white count with left shift, treatment should be immediate with parenteral antibiotics and close monitoring, preferably in a hospital setting. If there is difficulty with intravenous access, ceftriaxone 50 mg/kg can be given IM while access is being obtained.

Children who do not appear septic, in whom there is a low index of suspicion, and who are older than 2 years of age can be treated as outpatients with IM ceftriaxone while awaiting cultures, but **only if** close monitoring can be assured (daily evaluation and parents can be contacted by telephone). If all cultures are negative after 2 to 3 days and the child is afebrile and without symptoms, the antibiotics can be discontinued.

All patients who appear ill should be hospitalized and treated for presumed infection. Many children will develop increasing symptoms after being evaluated and hospitalized. ACS commonly occurs after hydration and is frequently precipitated by a vaso-occlusive pain episode.

VASO-OCCLUSIVE EPISODES

The bones and joints are the major sites of pain in sickle cell disease. In cancellous bones, such as the vertebrae, infarction can occur and eventually lead to collapse of the vertebral plates and compression. The classical radiographic appearance is of "fish mouth" disk spaces and the "step" sign (a depression in the central part of the vertebral body). Back pain is a common symptom in sickle cell disease, likely as a result of recurrent infarction and vertebral compression. Infarction in the long bones can cause swelling and edema in the overlying soft tissues. It may be difficult to differentiate a VOE from acute osteomyelitis. Although uncommon, infection should be considered. Osteomyelitis may be ruled out by close clinical observation, blood cultures, and, occasionally, aspiration of the affected area. Plain radiographs are not helpful in the early stages, and bone scans may not help differentiate a simple infarct from osteomyelitis.

Dactylitis, or hand–foot syndrome, refers to painful swelling of the hands and feet. This is seen exclusively in infants and young children (<5 years of age). It presents with pain, low-grade fever, and diffuse, nonpitting edema of the dorsum of the hands and feet that extends to the fingers. One or more extremities may be affected at a time. Radiographic changes (elevation of the periosteum of the phalanges or metatarsals) may appear 1 week or more after the clinical presentation. Therapy is with analgesics, hydration, and parental reassurance. Though the swelling and/or radiographic changes may persist for weeks, the syndrome is almost always self-limited. Transfusions and antibiotics are not necessary, unless there is concern for infection or the medical condition worsens.

Occasionally, there is a precipitating event that leads to the VOE: hypoxia (obstructive sleep apnea), fever, viral illness, or dehydration. There are a few children who have frequent pain episodes: It should not be taken for granted that each of these episodes is similar to the others, and a source for the painful event should be sought. If the pain changes or is very persistent, the child should be re-evaluated. If a young child has a symptom that is interpreted as pain, such as refusal to walk or a limp, also consider that the cause may be an acute central nervous system event.

The most common type of pain is **musculoskeletal pain**. The pain may be of any configuration: symmetric, migratory, or associated with erythema or swelling. There can be low-grade fevers, possibly associated with other clinical symptoms. It can sometimes be difficult to distinguish pain from infection, synovitis, or other pathologic processes.

Children are frequently seen with **abdominal pain**. A surgical abdominal problem needs to be considered. Children who have sickle cell anemia have a high incidence of cholecystitis. The differential should also consider pancreatitis, urinary tract infection, pelvic inflammatory disease, and pneumonia presenting as abdominal pain. Ileus and ACS are frequent complications of abdominal VOEs.

VOEs can last for many days. *Do not assume that the episode is controlled when the acute administration of analgesia is effective.* Children with these symptoms may have a medical problem that needs aggressive treatment beyond the therapy for their pain. A VOE is a diagnosis of exclusion. The pain needs to be treated while there is a work-up for cause of pain other than a VOE.

A reliable tool should be used to assess a child's level of pain. The assessment should be modified depending upon the age and developmental level of the child, and should be able to rate both subjective and objective aspects of the child's pain. Physicians should be familiar with the use of such assessment tools and refer to them when assessing children and adolescents who have pain.

High-risk factors for complications other than VOE in children with pain include the following:

- Fever greater than 101°F (38°C) orally and signs of infection
- Acute pulmonary symptoms (chest pain, hypoxia, abnormal auscultatory exam)
- Persistent vomiting
- Pain that is unusual for the patient
- Severe abdominal pain
- Extremity weakness or loss of function
- Any neurologic symptoms
- Severe headache
- Acute joint swelling

PAIN MANAGEMENT
Outpatient

Following are recommendations for the management of VOEs. However, many children and adolescents need individualized care plans for their routine treatment.

MILD PAIN
- Increase fluids to 1 to 1.25 times maintenance. Water, fruit juice, and fruit drinks as well as decaffeinated soda are recommended.
- Acetaminophen (15 mg/kg q4h) PO without codeine should be tried prior to using acetaminophen with codeine (1.0 mg/kg q4h). Many children do not take plain acetaminophen for vaso-occlusive pain.
- Ibuprofen (10 mg/kg q8h) PO should be used routinely, even if pain is temporarily controlled.
- Rest; heat to the area of pain
- Relaxation exercises, visualization, meditation

SEVERE PAIN
- IV hydration
  1. Bolus to correct fluid losses; then dextrose 5% in one-third normal saline (D_5 1/3 NS) IV at 1 to 1.25 times maintenance (IV + PO).
  2. Use caution not to overhydrate, especially if there are any pulmonary symptoms (overhydration can lead to pulmonary edema and precipitate ACS).

- Analgesics (IV)
  1. Morphine: 0.1 to 0.15 mg/kg/dose q3–4h. In children less than 2 years old who have not been exposed to narcotic analgesics, 0.1 mg/kg should be used.
  2. The pharmacokinetics of morphine differs between individual children, and doses must be titrated for individual patients.
  3. **Both underdosing and overdosing need to be avoided. Careful management is required!**

- Ketorolac (IV)
  1. Child: 1 mg/kg loading dose, then 0.5 mg/kg q6h
  2. Adult: 30 to 60 mg loading dose, then 15 to 30 mg q6h
  3. **Gastrointestinal bleeding** has been reported, so a histamine-2 blocker such as ranitidine is required if ketorolac is given IV. Morphine and ketorolac can be given simultaneously IM or in succession for the initial treatment of pain in children. Added to narcotic therapy, ketorolac increases analgesia and has a narcotic-sparing effect. Ketorolac is very useful in pain control, but should not be used in children for more than 5 days. There are numerous other analgesic medications that have been used to treat sickle cell pain.

GENERAL CONSIDERATIONS

Upon presentation to the clinic or emergency room, the child or adolescent should be rapidly assessed and treated for pain. Initially, both morphine and ketorolac should be given at the maximum recommended doses. If the pain returns, repeat the parenteral narcotic dose; it is unlikely oral analgesics will be successful if this regimen is not effective. If pain relief can be achieved and maintained for 3 hours, administer an oral narcotic and observe for 1 hour. If this regimen is successful, give a prescription for several days (10 to 15 doses) of narcotic and nonsteroidal anti-inflammatory medications. There should be follow-up within 72 hours. *If this regimen is not successful, or if other symptoms develop with hydration or a fever develops, the patient should be admitted for continued treatment and observation.*

Inpatient

As noted above, the administration of narcotics to acutely ill patients requires careful monitoring. A plan for pain management should be defined on admission and followed for the duration of hospitalization. In addition to whirlpool therapy, warm packs, and distraction therapy, routine care includes the following recommendations.

MANAGEMENT

- Correct fluid losses resulting from dehydration. Do not overhydrate children who have pulmonary symptoms.
- Total fluid intake (IV + PO) should be 1 to 1.25 times daily maintenance fluids.
- Monitor daily weight, obtain accurate input and output (I&O) record, and observe for signs of fluid overload.
- Encourage ambulation, sitting up in bed, and taking deep breaths.
- Institute incentive spirometry, 10 times an hour, every hour while awake.

ANALGESICS

- Pain medication should be administered on a fixed-time schedule, with an interval that does not extend beyond the duration of the analgesic effect. Do not give narcotics on a PRN basis except when the patient is ready for discharge.
- Titration schedules require a written plan, close observation, and a flow sheet to monitor effectiveness (sedation and hypoventilation can lead to hypoxia with resultant increased sickling and pain).
- **Patient-controlled analgesia** (PCA) is the method of choice for controlling pain in children who are 7 years of age or older. PCA protocols may be hospital specific. Generally, there is an initial bolus (0.1 mg/kg morphine), and an on-demand dose (0.01 to 0.04 mg/kg morphine) with a 10- to 20-minute lockout and a 1-hour maximum of 0.1 to 0.15 mg/kg of morphine. At night, there may be a need for a

continuous low-dose infusion (0.02 mg/kg/hr morphine) without changing the 1-hour lockout. Dilaudid is also an effective drug given by PCA.

GENERAL CONSIDERATIONS

Side effects of narcotics—respiratory depression, nausea, vomiting, pruritus, hypotension, constipation, inappropriate secretion of antidiuretic hormone, and change in seizure threshold—are accentuated in patients who take them for prolonged periods. Low-dose naloxone drip has been used for severe pruritus caused by morphine (see Formulary for dosing). The most common side effects of nausea, vomiting, and pruritus resolve over time. IV or PO diphenhydramine may be used safely in this setting. Meperidine should not be substituted for morphine. The metabolites of meperidine can accumulate and cause seizures, especially if used over a long period of time at high doses. A plan for withdrawal should be a part of discharge planning; clonidine hydrochloride has been used successfully for this purpose, but should be carefully monitored.

All patients who are hospitalized for pain should have **incentive spirometry at the bedside**. Ensure that the patient has been instructed on its use and can demonstrate appropriate use.

Alternative methods of pain control (behavior modification, relaxation, visualization, self-hypnosis, transcutaneous electrical nerve stimulation) are helpful adjuvants in the outpatient and inpatient settings but should not replace standard therapy. Children should have access to a psychologist who is experienced in the management of pain.

Drug addiction is extremely rare and should not be a primary concern. The goal should be to provide patients with adequate relief by understanding the pharmacology of the medications, drug tolerance, and physical dependence. Drug tolerance is common, and withdrawal symptoms after hospitalization are probably underreported by the patient. All patients should start a narcotic taper while in the hospital and complete this as an outpatient. On average, patients admitted for management of VOE require 3 to 7 days of inpatient care.

ACUTE CHEST SYNDROME/PNEUMONIA

ACS is defined as the development of a new pulmonary infiltrate in the presence of fever or respiratory symptoms. Because chest radiograph changes may be delayed, the diagnosis may not be apparent at presentation. Approximately 50% of children who have sickle cell disease will have ACS. ACS is frequently caused by community-acquired pathogens such as *Chlamydia, Mycoplasma*, and other bacterial or viral organisms. In older children, adolescents, and young adults, ACS may be more commonly associated with vaso-occlusion, infarction, fat embolism, or in situ sickling. These episodes are characterized by chest pain, fever, hypoxia, and pulmonary infiltrates. Though ACS usually improves with medical management, it can present with or progress rapidly to respiratory failure (adult respiratory distress syndrome), requiring mechanical ventilation and emergent blood transfusion or exchange.

Sixty percent of children who have pneumonia on chest radiograph will be missed by physical exam alone. Many children who have a negative chest film on admission will develop findings after hydration. All children who have symptoms of pulmonary disease, such as fever, shortness of breath, tachypnea, chest pain, cough, wheezing, rales, or dullness to percussion, should have an assessment of oxygen saturation and a chest radiograph, receive parenteral antibiotics, and be admitted to the hospital. Bronchodilators and incentive spirometry are helpful adjuncts in treatment and prevention of worsening ACS. If there is an infiltrate, the patient should be closely observed for hypoxia and progression of pulmonary infiltrates, with repeat chest radiographs. Overhydration can lead to pulmonary edema and exacerbate ACS. Oversedation with narcotics can also lead to hypoventilation, increasing the risk for ACS. Narcotics should be used with caution in this setting.

ACS can develop in a matter of hours and is associated with a high rate of morbidity and mortality. Children should have oxygen saturation monitored and, if indicated, arterial blood gases should be determined. Oxygen therapy should be used only for hypoxia documented by a blood gas measurement. Supplemental oxygen can decrease erythropoietin production and lead to more severe anemia. Pulmonary infections should be treated aggressively, and these children watched closely. If there is no improvement, a red blood cell transfusion (straight or exchange, dependent upon the severity of the hypoxia and anemia and clinical status of the patient) may help to correct the anemia, decrease the percentage of Hgb S, and improve oxygen-carrying capacity to aid in reversing the pulmonary sickling and improving the clinical course. Transfusions are more effective when administered early in the course of ACS, rather than as a life-saving measure in a critically ill child.

There is a distinct difference between the etiology of ACS in children versus adolescents and adults. In children, the incidence of ACS is seasonal, lower in the summer months with increasing rates in the winter when viral infections are prevalent.

In adults and adolescents, ACS is frequently a complication of an episode of vaso-occlusion (without fever) caused by pulmonary fat embolism. This event will progress to include chest pain and fever and a pulmonary infiltrate, usually basilar with pleural effusion. Adults and adolescents more frequently need transfusions and less frequently have a viral or bacterial infection associated with their episode of ACS. Individuals who have Hgb SC have relatively more fat in their marrow and can actually have more severe pulmonary fat emboli when their course is complicated by ACS.

3

ACUTE CHEST SYNDROME/PNEUMONIA

Stroke and other central nervous system events are more common in children who have ACS within the 2-week period after the event.

LABORATORY EVALUATION OF ACUTE CHEST SYNDROME

- CBC and reticulocyte count, manual differential
- Type and hold blood for possible transfusion
- Chest radiograph, as often as clinically indicated to monitor progression of disease
- Continuous pulse oximetry and baseline arterial blood gas (on room air if possible)
- Blood culture for fever
- Phospholipase A_2 is being evaluated as an indicator of impending ACS and is usually elevated 24 to 48 hours prior to the development of ACS. This study is dependent on institution availability.

MANAGEMENT

All patients with evidence of acute pulmonary pathology should be admitted to the hospital. If fever is present or if an infectious process is suspected, antibiotic therapy should be started immediately (Fig. 3–2).

- Oxygen
  1. Hypoxemic patients (p_aO_2 <70 to 80 mm Hg, O_2 saturation 90% to 95%): 2 L/minute by nasal cannula.
  2. Re-evaluate arterial blood gas on oxygen.

- Antibiotics
  1. Initiate broad-spectrum antibiotic such as cefuroxime 150 mg/kg/day IV divided q8h, after cultures are obtained (adults 2.5 to 4.5 g/day, maximum 2 g/dose).
  2. Because of the frequency of atypical organisms (*Chlamydia, Mycoplasma*), a macrolide or quinolone antibiotic should be included, such as erythromycin at a dose of 50 mg/kg/day divided q6–8h (adults: maximum 4 g/day divided q6h).

- Analgesics: as indicated for vaso-occlusive pain management. Administration must be monitored to provide the maximum pain control and prevent hypoventilation or atelectasis due to splinting or narcotization.
- Hydration PO + IV hydration (D_5 1/3 NS); limit to 1.25 times maintenance fluids. Caution should be used in patients with potential ACS to avoid fluid overload. Monitor I&O, daily weight.
- Other supportive measures
  1. Continuous pulse oximetry
  2. Incentive spirometry, 10 times an hour, every hour while awake (prevention of hypoventilation)
  3. Albuterol aerosols q4h (airway hyper-reactivity is common in ACS)

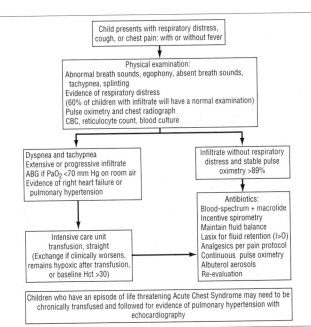

FIGURE 3–2

Approach to acute pulmonary infiltrate in a child with sickle cell disease. (Abbreviations: CBC = complete blood count; ABG = arterial blood gas; Hct = hematocrit; I&O = input and output.)

- Physical therapy
  1. Warm packs
  2. Ambulation as tolerated, sitting up in bed

- Transfusion
  1. Straight transfusion
  2. Exchange transfusion (for patients with hematocrit >30)
  3. Transfusion decreases the proportion of sickling red cells and increases blood oxygen affinity. The main indication is worsening respiratory function, as documented by hypoxemia (p_aO_2 <70 mm Hg on room air), worsening chest pain, evolving clinical examination, or worsening infiltrates on chest radiograph. For patients with chronic hypoxemia, a drop of greater than 10% of baseline is a reasonable level at which to transfuse. Delays in instituting transfusion therapy, particularly in rapidly deteriorating patients, should be avoided.

PRIAPISM

Forty percent of men who are homozygous for Hgb S report having priapism in their adolescence and early adulthood. Priapism has a second peak at 21 to 29 years. Priapism is defined as a painful erection that lasts for more than 30 minutes. It frequently results in interference with the urinary stream. Priapism can be precipitated by prolonged intercourse or masturbation; it frequently occurs at night and can be differentiated from a nocturnal erection by its duration and pain. Children will occasionally complain of dysuria as the first complaint of priapism. Prognosis is poorer in adolescents and adults who have recurrent prolonged priapism, and, if aggressive treatment is not successful, impotence may result. Children who have priapism generally have a better prognosis and usually do not have prolonged priapism requiring aggressive therapy. Priapism can occur with VOEs and with fever and sepsis.

Priapism can occur as a sudden severe episode of painful erection that can last for hours, days, or weeks with moderate to severe pain, or it can occur as a pattern of painful erections that recur over a period of days or several weeks (stuttering priapism). Chronic nonpainful priapism can also occur.

Because priapism can lead to impotence, early medical management is indicated. A urologist who is familiar with priapism in sickle cell disease should be consulted. Treatment includes hydration, exchange transfusion, intracavernous injection of α-adrenergic agents, and shunting surgery. Oral α-adrenergics (pseudoephedrine hydrochloride 30 mg BID) have been used successfully to treat stuttering priapism. Chronic transfusion therapy has been used in patients with recurrent priapism (maintenance of Hgb S below 30%), though no controlled trials have been performed proving the efficacy of this therapy.

STROKE (CEREBROVASCULAR ACCIDENT)

Stroke is a common event in children homozygous for Hgb S. **Between 10% and 15% of children with sickle cell disease suffer from overt strokes.** In children, strokes are more frequently the result of cerebral vascular stenosis and infarction. The mean age of occurrence of clinically evident stroke is 7 to 8 years, with the highest risk occurring between 2 and 9 years. Hemorrhage and infarct may occur together.

Strokes in children who have sickle cell disease involve stenosis and occlusion of the major anterior arteries of the brain, including the carotids. The **presenting symptoms of stroke** can be dramatic and acute, such as coma, seizure, hemiparesis, hemianesthesia, visual field deficits, aphasia, or cranial nerve palsies. Subtle limb weakness (without pain) is often mistaken for an acute VOE but can be due to stroke. Classically, the symptoms must persist for 24 hours. The presentation of severe headache and vomiting with no other neurologic findings can be symptomatic of an intracranial hemorrhage.

Initially, a computed tomography (CT) scan without contrast will be normal for up to 6 hours after a stroke but will rule out intracerebral hemorrhage, abscess, tumor, or other pathology that would explain the neurologic symptoms. Magnetic resonance imaging (MRI) and magnetic resonance angiography (MRA) are much more sensitive methods to determine intracranial infarct but can remain normal for 2 to 4 hours after an event. All catastrophic neurologic events should first be evaluated with CT because it is generally more available and will rule out acute pathology. Cerebral arteriography should be obtained to document abnormalities seen on MRA.

Initially, even prior to definitive diagnosis and imaging, children are **exchange transfused** to a Hgb S of less than 30%. Blood pressure should be continually monitored during an exchange transfusion, bearing in mind that, relative to the normal population, children with sickle cell disease are hypotensive. The diagnosis of stroke in children can be made on clinical findings and treated emergently. Children should be monitored until they are stable and the hemoglobin electrophoresis is documented. Those who have had a stroke require chronic transfusion therapy for an undetermined length of time.

Children with sickle cell disease have more frequent and more severe **headaches** than other children; these may be the manifestation of cerebral hypoxia and vasodilatation. Children who have severe headaches accompanied by vomiting need extensive evaluation with imaging, neurologic testing, and neuropsychological testing.

Transcranial Doppler (TCD) has been shown to predict increased risk of stroke in children who have increased flow velocity in major cerebral arteries. Unsuspected cerebral vascular damage was detected by CT and MRI in 25% to 30% of children in the Cooperative Study of Sickle Cell Disease, but no clinical factors, with the exception of TCD, predicted the occurrence of stroke. In this study there was a correlation between first stroke and transient ischemic attack, ACS, elevated systolic blood pressure, and severe anemia. All children who can cooperate with TCD (usually by 2 years of age) should have an annual evaluation if the study is available locally. Normal middle cerebral artery velocity in children with sickle cell disease is approximately 120 cm/second. Children who have velocities of 170 to 199 cm/second are considered high risk, and those with velocities of 200 cm/second or higher are even higher risk. The recent STOP trial (Stroke Prevention Trial in Sickle Cell Anemia) showed that transfusion greatly reduces the risk of a first stroke in children who have abnormally high (velocity >200 cm/second) results on TCD. Prophylactic chronic transfusions are often started if there are two studies at least 2 weeks apart with velocities greater than 200 cm/second. Compliance issues and risks of chronic transfusions must also be considered when deciding on this therapy.

Transient ischemic attacks are defined as a focal neurologic deficit with a vascular distribution persisting for fewer than 48 hours. These patients are treated in a manner similar to those who have an infarct. The diagnosis is made in retrospect when the follow-up MRI is negative for a persistent lesion that would explain the neurologic symptoms.

Intracerebral hemorrhage or **subarachnoid hemorrhage** may present without focal neurologic symptoms. Exchange transfusion should be carried out immediately. Arteriography is used to identify the arterial bleed, and the patient may need emergent surgical intervention. Mortality is very high during the acute event (50%).

ACUTE ANEMIA

There are two common causes of acute life-threatening anemia in sickle cell disease: splenic sequestration and aplastic crisis.

SPLENIC SEQUESTRATION

Infants and young children who have Hgb SS or $S\beta^0$ thalassemia and older children (over 10 years) who have Hgb SC or $S\beta^+$ syndromes can have intrasplenic pooling of large amounts of blood and platelets. This can lead to anemia, thrombocytopenia, hypovolemia, cardiovascular collapse, and sudden death within hours of the onset of sequestration. The syndrome has been reported in infants as young as 2 months of age. Classically, however, it occurs from after the disappearance of Hgb F, at about 5 to 6 months of age, to approximately 3 years of age in children with Hgb SS when the spleen becomes fibrotic as a result of multiple infarctions. These crises can occur in **older** children who have Hgb SC or $S\beta^+$ but are usually not as severe; still, fatal events have been recorded for these children. The incidence is between 10% and 30% and the recurrence rate is 50%. Mild events can indicate the possibility of life-threatening sequestration events. Chronic sequestration can also be a sequela, with chronic anemia and thrombocytopenia.

The clinical presentation is usually rapid in onset. Usually the child will have sudden weakness, pallor of the lips and mucous membranes, breathlessness, rapid pulse, faintness, and abdominal fullness. Evaluation of the CBC will frequently show a precipitous drop from the baseline hemoglobin.

The **treatment** for splenic sequestration is transfusion to restore circulating blood volume, usually with phenotypically matched blood (unless there is a life-threatening situation). As the shock is reversed and the transfused blood decreases the percentage of Hgb S, the splenomegaly regresses, and much of the blood is remobilized with a rapid rise in the child's hemoglobin.

Splenectomy should be strongly considered in all children who have a splenic sequestration crisis. Transfusions can prevent recurrence until surgery can be arranged. Some children who have Hgb SS and older children who have other S hemoglobinopathies can have massive splenomegaly with **hypersplenism** after an episode of splenic sequestration. If hypersplenism (anemia, neutropenia and/or thrombocytopenia) is persistent and severe, splenectomy is indicated.

Prior to splenectomy, younger children should have an evaluation of splenic function with a **pit count** and a spleen scan. In normally eusplenic persons, fewer than 1% of the circulating red cells are pitted; values of 2% to 12% may represent decreased splenic function. If the child still has a functional spleen, usually under 2 years of age, a partial splenectomy can be performed. Children should have appropriate immunizations, including pneumococcal vaccination, prior to splenectomy. **Penicillin** prophylaxis is continued indefinitely in **all** children who have been splenectomized.

APLASTIC CRISIS

Severe anemia can develop over several days as a result of shortened red cell survival without compensatory reticulocytosis. Reticulocytopenia can last 7 to 10 days. The primary cause of transient red cell aplasia is parvovirus B19, though it can follow other viral infections as well. **Parvovirus B19, the most common cause of aplasia in children with hemoglobinopathies,** can also cause neutropenia. Although many patients recover spontaneously, the anemia can be profound. Red cell transfusions are indicated for those who become symptomatic of the anemia or if the hemoglobin falls below 2 g/dl from their baseline. Symptoms occurring with aplastic crisis include nausea and vomiting, myalgias, and arthralgias. Splenic and hepatic sequestration have also been reported with aplastic crises. If it is thought that the child will not be able to return for evaluation, then the child should be hospitalized for observation. The patient should be isolated from other patients with chronic hemolytic anemias (sickle cell disease or thalassemia) or red cell aplasia and should not have pregnant caregivers. If the child is mildly anemic and asymptomatic, outpatient monitoring is reasonable.

AVASCULAR NECROSIS

Bone pain is common in sickle cell disease. Marrow infarcts can cause pain that can last for weeks. Avascular necrosis (osteonecrosis) causes pain that can sometimes be confused with a bone infarct. Symptoms of avascular necrosis, such as limping, can sometimes be confused with stroke. Limping with weakness is indicative of stroke, not avascular necrosis.

Avascular necrosis is common in all age groups, but is more frequently diagnosed in the adolescent, and involves the humeral and femoral heads. It is more common in individuals who have Hgb $S\beta^0$ thalassemia and Hgb SS with α-thalassemia. It is also seen, though with a lower frequency, in those who have Hgb $S\beta^+$ thalassemia. Individuals who have Hgb SS are more frequently affected than those with Hgb SC.

Avascular necrosis is a result of an infarct in the cancellous trabeculae in the head of either the femur or the humerus. The process of necrosis and repair can be progressive, leading to collapse of the head, or there can be arrest with varying degrees of disability and sclerosis. Listed below is a method of describing the progression of avascular necrosis:

Stage 0: no evidence of disease
Stage 1: Radiograph normal, bone scan abnormal, MRI abnormal
Stage 2: Radiograph shows sclerosis and cystic changes without collapse
Stage 3: Subchondral collapse (crescent sign) without collapse
Stage 4: Collapse and flattening of the femoral head without acetabular involvement, normal joint space
Stage 5: Joint narrowing and/or acetabular involvement
Stage 6: Increased joint narrowing and/or acetabular involvement

Treatment for avascular necrosis of the femur includes bed rest with crutch walking for 6 weeks, nonsteroidal anti-inflammatory medication, and core decompression surgery for stages 1 or 2. The surgery is relatively simple; a core is removed from the head of the femur. The coring begins approximately 2 cm below the trochanteric ridge, extending through the neck and into the head of the femur. Acutely, this procedure provides relief of pain and is thought to arrest the progression of avascular necrosis, though this has not been confirmed in a prospective trial.

RETINOPATHY/HYPHEMA

The eye is particularly sensitive to hypoxia. Vaso-occlusion of retinal vessels and hypoxia of the retina causes permanent retinal damage. Blood in the anterior chamber of the eye (hyphema) becomes rapidly deoxygenated and permanently sickled, obstructing the outflow from the aqueous humor. The accumulation of aqueous humor in the anterior chamber increases intraocular pressure, leading to decreased blood flow in the retina until the perfusion pressure of the globe is reached. This leads to sudden vascular stasis and blindness. The events occurring in hyphema can also occur in children who have sickle cell trait.

Retinal vascular occlusion initially occurs in peripheral retinal vessels without significant sequelae. It eventually leads to neovascularization from the retina into the vitreous (sea fans). These abnormal vessels are fragile and can bleed into the vitreous, causing "floaters" or blindness if the hemorrhage is sufficient. If bleeds do not obscure vision and are unnoticed, they can cause collapse of the vitreous, traction on the retina, and eventually retinal detachment. Retinal disease of the eye is common in sickle cell disease. It occurs most commonly in individuals who have Hgb SC.

Treatment of sickle cell **retinopathy** requires recognition. The damaged peripheral vessels are not generally appreciated by direct ophthalmic examination and require the use of an indirect binocular stereoscopic ophthalmoscope. Sea fanning, vitreous hemorrhage, and detachment can be observed by direct ophthalmoscopy. Annual ophthalmic evaluations should begin at age 10 for all children who have sickle cell disease. Treatment of early neovascularization requires laser photocoagulation. Surgical approaches are required for advanced lesions.

Hyphema is a medical emergency in sickle cell disease. It requires immediate ophthalmic evaluation and transfusion (exchange or straight) to reduce sickling and improve oxygenation. If a conservative approach is not successful, anterior chamber paracentesis is performed to relieve intraocular pressure and remove the hyphema.

HYPERBILIRUBINEMIA/GALLSTONES

Bilirubin gallstones can eventually be detected in most patients with a chronic hemolytic anemia. In sickle cell disease, gallstones occur in children as young as 3 to 4 years of age, and are eventually found in approximately 70% of patients. It may be difficult to differentiate between gallbladder disease and abdominal vaso-occlusive crisis in patients with recurrent abdominal pain. Cholecystectomy may be necessary for patients with fat intolerance, presence of gallstones, and recurrent abdominal pain.

Hepatomegaly and liver dysfunction may be caused by a combination of intrahepatic trapping of sickled cells, transfusion-acquired infection, and/or transfusional hemosiderosis. The combination of hemolysis, liver dysfunction, and renal tubular defects can result in very high bilirubin levels. Benign cholestasis of sickle cell disease results in severe asymptomatic hyperbilirubinemia without fever, pain, leukocytosis, or hepatic failure.

PERIOPERATIVE CARE FOR SICKLE CELL PATIENTS

Careful management is necessary for sickle cell patients who have surgical procedures or require anesthesia for other purposes. General anesthesia results in atelectasis and hypoxia, which are not otherwise tolerated if the patient is significantly anemic, and special precautions must be taken perioperatively to decrease morbidity and mortality associated with even minor surgical procedures. Other risk factors include the presence of chronic organ damage in some patients, the effects of asplenia, and the propensity for the sickle cells to sickle and obstruct microvasculature as a result of even mild hypoxia. The guidelines suggested below are extrapolated from a multicenter randomized trial of transfusion (exchange versus straight) in the perioperative period.

PREOPERATIVE CARE

1. Admission to the hospital the afternoon prior to the scheduled surgery
2. Hydration at 1.25 to 1.5 times maintenance (IV + PO) beginning the evening and night prior to surgery
3. Pulse oximetry on room air (spot checks)
4. Incentive spirometry at least 10 times per hour while awake

5. Lab work: CBC with differential and reticulocyte count, urinalysis, type and cross, chemistry panel
6. Transfusion: All sickle cell patients should have a **red cell phenotype** study obtained prior to any transfusion. Sickle cell patients should receive partially phenotypically matched blood to decrease the risk of alloimmunization. In addition, all blood should be Sickledex negative and leukodepleted. The following transfusion guidelines are recommended (see also Chapter 5):
   a. Patients with Hgb SS or $S\beta^0$ disease who are undergoing any procedure other than myringotomy tube placement should have a simple transfusion to achieve a hemoglobin of 10 to 12 g/dl. Do not exceed 12 g/dl because of the risk of stasis/sludging.
   b. Patients with Hgb SC disease or $S\beta^+$ who have baseline hemoglobins below 10 g/dl may at times need transfusions to achieve a hemoglobin of 10 to 12 g/dl. However, **DO NOT** transfuse these patients prior to consulting the hematologist. Many factors may affect this decision, including a history of significant complications of their sickle cell disease (pneumonia, VOEs, priapism, aseptic necrosis, etc.). Consult the hematologist if there is confusion regarding individual patients.
7. Patients with central venous catheters or those undergoing dental procedures should receive antibiotic prophylaxis prior to surgery.

POSTOPERATIVE CARE

1. Adequate pain management to prevent splinting and atelectasis, with care to prevent narcosis
2. Pulse oximetry for at least the first 12 to 24 hours postoperatively
3. Continuous oxygen 1 to 2 L by nasal cannula for at least the first 12 to 24 hours postoperatively
4. Incentive spirometry at least 10 times per hour while awake. Be aggressive!
5. Ambulation as early as possible, taking into account the specific surgical procedures
6. Lab work: CBC with reticulocyte count q_{AM}
7. Follow-up in clinic approximately 1 week after hospital discharge or sooner if there are ongoing problems

TRANSFUSION THERAPY

Red blood cell transfusion increases oxygen-carrying capacity and improves microvascular perfusion by decreasing the proportion of sickled red cells. Transfusions are given to patients with sickle cell disease to stabilize or reverse an acute medical complication, or as part of chronic therapy in certain situations to prevent future complications.

INDICATIONS
Acute Illnesses
1. Splenic sequestration
2. Transient red cell aplasia
3. Hyperhemolysis (infection, ACS)

Patients should be transfused if there is evidence of cardiovascular compromise (heart failure, dyspnea, hypertension, or marked fatigue). Generally, transfusion is indicated if the hemoglobin falls below 5 g/dl or drops below 2 g/dl from the steady state.

Sudden Severe Illness
1. Acute chest syndrome
2. Stroke
3. Sepsis
4. Acute multiorgan failure

These life-threatening illnesses are often accompanied by a falling hemoglobin. Transfusion therapy has become standard medical practice in the management of these illnesses. When ACS is associated with hypoxia and a falling hemoglobin, transfusion is indicated. Many patients can be treated with straight transfusion, though, in severe cases, exchange transfusion or red cell pheresis is recommended. Studies suggest that early transfusion may prevent progression of acute pulmonary disease.

The efficacy of transfusion in the management of acute stroke has not been well studied, though anecdotal reports indicate early exchange transfusion may limit neuronal damage by improving local oxygenation and perfusion. Chronic transfusion therapy reduces the rate of recurrence and is indicated in all patients after a first stroke.

PERIOPERATIVE TRANSFUSION
Patients with sickle cell anemia undergoing major surgery should be prepared in advance by transfusion to a hemoglobin of approximately 10 g/dl and a decrease in hemoglobin S percentage to approximately 60%. While standard practice guidelines have not been developed for Hgb SS patients undergoing minor procedures or for surgery in those with Hgb SC, it is generally acceptable to not transfuse these patients, assuming they are medically stable.

CHRONIC TRANSFUSION THERAPY
Chronic transfusions are indicated in several conditions in which the potential medical complications warrant the risks of alloimmunization, infection, and transfusional iron overload. Transfusions are given every 3 to 4 weeks, with a goal to maintain the hemoglobin S at 30% to 50%. Although straight transfusions are acceptable, red cell pheresis or exchange transfusions may be preferred to decrease the rate of iron overload.

Indications
1. Primary stroke prevention
2. Pulmonary hypertension/chronic lung disease
3. Chronic debilitating pain

Transfusions are sometimes suggested for a number of conditions in which efficacy is unproven, but may be considered under severe circumstances. Such circumstances include

1. Acute priapism
2. Pregnancy (frequent complications)
3. "Silent" cerebral infarcts
4. Leg ulcers

SUGGESTED READING

Adams RJ, McKie VC, Hsu L, et al. Prevention of a first stroke by transfusions in children with sickle cell anemia and abnormal results on transcranial Doppler ultrasonography. N Engl J Med 339:5–11, 1998.

Bruno D, Wigfall DR, Zimmerman SA. Genitourinary complications of sickle cell disease. J Urol 166:803–811, 2001.

Charache S, Lubin B, Reid CD (eds). Management and Therapy of Sickle Cell Disease. Washington, DC: National Institutes of Health, 1989.

Golden C, Styles L, Vichinsky E. Acute chest syndrome and sickle cell disease. Curr Opin Hematol 5:89–92, 1998.

Morris C, Vichinsky E, Styles L. Clinician assessment for acute chest syndrome in febrile patients with sickle cell disease: is it accurate enough? Ann Emerg Med 34: 64–69, 1999.

Reed W, Vichinsky EP. Transfusion therapy: a coming-of-age treatment for patients with sickle cell disease. J Pediatr Hematol Oncol 23:197–202, 2001.

THALASSEMIA

The thalassemias are a diverse group of genetic diseases characterized by absent or decreased production of normal hemoglobin, resulting in a microcytic anemia (Table 4–1). The α-thalassemias are concentrated in Southeast Asia, Malaysia, and Southern China. The β-thalassemias are seen primarily in the Mediterranean, Africa, and Southeast Asia. As a result of global migration patterns, there is an increase in the incidence of thalassemia in North America, primarily because of immigration from Southeast Asia.

Normally, 95% of adult hemoglobin found on electrophoresis is Hgb A ($\alpha^2\beta^2$). Two minor hemoglobins occur: 2% to 3.5% is Hgb A$_2$ ($\alpha^2\delta^2$), and less than 2% is Hgb F ($\alpha^2\gamma^2$). A mutation affecting globin chain production or deletion of one of the globin chains leads to a decreased production of that chain and an abnormal globin ratio. The globin that is produced in normal amounts is in excess and forms red cell aggregates or inclusions. These aggregates become oxidized and damage the cell membrane, leading to ineffective erythropoiesis, hemolysis, or both. The quantity and properties of these globin chain aggregates determine the phenotypic characteristics of the thalassemia.

An excess of α-globin chains (β-thalassemia) leads to formation of α-globin tetramers that accumulate in the erythroblast. These aggregates are very insoluble, and their precipitation interferes with erythropoiesis, cell maturation, and cell membrane function, leading to ineffective erythropoiesis and anemia.

An excess of β-globin chains (α-thalassemia) leads to tetramers of β-globin (Hgb H). These tetramers are more stable and soluble as the red cell ages in the circulation, and, under conditions of oxidant stress, Hgb H precipitates and interferes with membrane function, leading to an increase in hemolysis.

α-THALASSEMIA

The α-thalassemias are caused by a decrease in production of α-globin due to a deletion or mutation of one or more of the four α-globin genes located on chromosome 16. Alpha gene mapping can be obtained to determine the specific mutation. The α-thalassemias can be generally categorized as silent carrier, α-thalassemia trait, hemoglobin H disease, hemoglobin H–Constant Spring, and α-thalassemia major (Table 4–2). Frequently, the diagnosis of α-thalassemia trait in a parent is discovered after the birth of an affected child.

SILENT CARRIER
Silent carrier status is characterized by three functional genes for α-globin ($-\alpha/\alpha\alpha$). Outside the newborn period, it is not possible to make this diagnosis by conventional methods. There is overlap between the red blood cell

TABLE 4–1

CLASSIFICATION OF THE THALASSEMIAS

Silent Carrier	Hematologically normal
Thalassemia Trait (α-thalassemia trait or β-thalassemia trait)	Mild anemia with microcytosis and hypochromia
Hemoglobin H Disease (α-thalassemia) *or*	Moderately severe hemolytic anemia
Hemoglobin H–Constant Spring	Icterus and splenomegaly
Thalassemia Major	Severe anemia, hepatosplenomegaly
Thalassemia Intermedia	Some features of thalassemia major without regular transfusion requirement

indices of these individuals and normal persons, although the mean cell volume may be slightly lower. This state is deduced when a "normal" individual has a child with Hgb H disease or with microcytic anemia consistent with α-thalassemia trait. An unusual case of the silent carrier state is the individual who carries the hemoglobin Constant Spring mutation ($\alpha_{cs}\alpha/\alpha\alpha$ or $\alpha\alpha_{cs}/\alpha\alpha$). This is an elongated α-globin resulting from a termination codon mutation. Individuals who have this mutation have normal red blood cell indices, but can have children who have Hgb H–Constant Spring if the other parent has α-thalassemia trait ($\alpha\alpha/{-\!-}$). Generally these children are more affected clinically than other children who have Hgb H.

TABLE 4–2

α-THALASSEMIA SYNDROMES

SYNDROME*	CLINICAL FINDINGS	HEMOGLOBINS
Silent Carrier (1-gene deletion)	No anemia, normal- appearing red cells	1%–2% Hgb Bart's (γ^4) at birth; may have 1%–2% Hgb CS[†]
α-Thalassemia Trait (2-gene deletion)	Mild anemia, hypochromic- and microcytic-appearing red cells	5%– 10% Hgb Bart's (γ^4) at birth; may have 1%– 2% Hgb CS,[†] 80%–95% Hgb A
Hemoglobin H Disease (3-gene deletion)	Moderate anemia; frag- mented hypochromic and microcytic red cells; red cell inclu- sions	5%– 30% Hgb Bart's (γ^4) at birth; may have 1%– 2% Hgb CS,[†] 70%– 90% Hgb A

*A 4-gene deletion is not generally considered compatible with life (hydrops fetalis).
[†]Hgb CS = Hemoglobin Constant Spring.

α-THALASSEMIA TRAIT

Individuals who have α-thalassemia trait (−α/−α or αα/—) are identified by microcytosis, erythrocytosis, hypochromia, and mild anemia. The diagnosis is made by family studies, ruling out both iron deficiency anemia and β-thalassemia trait. In the neonatal period, when hemoglobin Bart's (γ^4) is present, the diagnosis can be suspected. In children there are no markers such as elevated Hgb A_2 and Hgb F (seen in β-thalassemia trait) to make the diagnosis. The diagnosis is one of exclusion. During pregnancy, the microcytic anemia can be mistaken for anemia of pregnancy.

HEMOGLOBIN H

Hemoglobin H (—/−α) should be considered in the case of a neonate in whom all of the red blood cells are very hypochromic. Neonates who have Hgb H will also have a high percentage of Hgb Bart's on their newborn screen. In children, this hemoglobinopathy is characterized by moderate anemia with a hemoglobin in the 8- to 10-g/dl range, hypochromia, microcytosis, red cell fragmentation, and a fast-migrating hemoglobin (Hgb H) on electrophoresis.

Hemoglobin H does not function as a normal hemoglobin and has a high oxygen affinity, so the measured hemoglobin in these children is misleading. Individuals who have Hgb H generally have a persistent stable state of anemia that may be accentuated by increased hemolysis during viral infections and by exposure to oxidant medications, chemicals, and foods (e.g., sulfa drugs, benzene, and fava beans), similar to individuals who have glucose-6-phosphate dehydrogenase deficiency. As the red cells mature, they lose their ability to withstand oxidant stress and Hgb H precipitates, leading to hemolysis. Therapy for individuals who have Hgb H disease includes folate, avoidance of oxidant drugs and foods, genetic counseling, education, and frequent medical care. Uncommon occurrences in a child with Hgb H would be severe anemia, cholelithiasis, skin ulceration, and splenomegaly requiring splenectomy. Unlike individuals who have β-thalassemia, hemosiderosis is rare in Hgb H disease.

HEMOGLOBIN H–CONSTANT SPRING

Children with hemoglobin H–Constant Spring (—/α$_{cs}$α) have a more severe course than children who have Hgb H. They have a more severe anemia, with a steady-state hemoglobin ranging between 7 and 8 g/dl. They more frequently have splenomegaly and severe anemia with febrile illnesses and viral infections, often requiring transfusion. If anemia is chronically severe and the child has splenomegaly, a splenectomy may be performed. *A complication can be severe postsplenectomy thrombocytosis with hypercoagulability, leading to thrombosis of the splenic vein or hepatic veins.* This complication has also been reported as recurrent pulmonary emboli and clotting diathesis. If splenectomy is anticipated, children who are scheduled to have surgery are treated with low-molecular-weight heparin, followed by low-dose aspirin, continued indefinitely.

α-THALASSEMIA MAJOR

The most severe form of α-thalassemia is α-thalassemia major (—/—). This diagnosis is frequently made in the last months of pregnancy when fetal ultrasound indicates a hydropic fetus. The mothers frequently exhibit toxemia and can develop severe postpartum hemorrhage. These infants are usually stillborn. There can be other congenital anomalies, though none are pathognomonic for α-thalassemia major. As a result of in utero hypoxia, the hemoglobins found in these infants are Hgb Portland ($\zeta^2\gamma^2$), Hgb H (β^4), and Hgb Bart's (γ^4), and no Hgb A or A$_2$. These babies can have other complications associated with hydrops, such as heart failure and pulmonary edema. If the diagnosis is made early, intrauterine transfusions can be performed. There are reports of survival and chronic transfusion in these infants. Bone marrow transplant from a matched sibling donor is potentially curative. Undoubtedly, more of these infants could be saved if the condition was anticipated by prenatal diagnosis and treatment provided.

β-THALASSEMIA

The β- and α-thalassemias have a distribution similar to that of areas where *Plasmodium falciparum* malaria is common. There are hundreds of mutations within the β-globin gene, but about 20 different alleles make up about 80% of the mutations found worldwide. Within each geographic population there are unique mutations. Individuals who have β-thalassemia major are usually homozygous for one of the common mutations and one of the geographically unique mutations that lead to absence of beta chain production.

The β-thalassemia syndromes are much more diverse than the α-thalassemia syndromes because of the diversity of the mutations that produce the defects in the β-globin gene. Unlike the deletions that constitute most of the α-thalassemia syndromes, β-thalassemias are caused by mutations on chromosome 11 that affect all aspects of β-globin production: transcription, translation, and the stability of the β-globin product. Most hematologists believe there are three general categories of β-thalassemia: β-thalassemia trait, thalassemia intermedia, and β-thalassemia major.

Splice-site mutations also occur and are of clinical consequence, when combined with a thalassemia mutation. Three splice-site mutations occur in exon 1 of the β-globin gene. These mutations result in three different abnormal hemoglobins: Malay, E, and Knossos. **Hemoglobin E** is a very common abnormal hemoglobin in the Southeast Asian population and, when paired with a β^0 thalassemia mutation, can produce severe transfusion-dependent thalassemia.

β-THALASSEMIA TRAIT

Individuals who have β-thalassemia trait have microcytosis and hypochromia; there may be targeting and elliptocytosis, though some individuals have an almost normal smear. These hematologic features can be accentuated in women with β-thalassemia trait who are pregnant and individuals who are folate or iron deficient. If iron deficiency is concurrent with β-thalassemia trait, there may be a normal Hgb A_2. Iron deficiency causes decreased β-thalassemia hemoglobin production, and folate or vitamin B_{12} deficiency can lead to megaloblastic anemia with increased Hgb A_2. Both of these deficiencies need to be treated prior to evaluation for thalassemia trait. In iron-, B_{12}-, and folate-replete individuals, the Hgb A_2 can be as high as 3.5% to 8% and the Hgb F as high as 1% to 5%. Generally, β-thalassemia trait is milder in African-Americans (who frequently have a promoter gene mutation) but has a similar presentation in individuals of Chinese, Southeast Asian, Greek, Italian, and Middle Eastern heritage.

Infants born in most states in the United States are screened for hemoglobinopathies. In states without newborn screening for hemoglobinopathies and in recent immigrants to this country, affected children are frequently found later than the newborn period, and the evaluation of their microcytic anemia includes differentiation between iron deficiency and β-thalassemia trait. The red blood cell indices can be helpful in this differentiation because the hemoglobin concentration and the red cell count will generally be lower in iron deficiency. The distinguishing finding in β-thalassemia is a hemoglobin electrophoresis with the finding of elevated Hgb A_2 and F. Both will be increased in β-thalassemia trait without iron deficiency, and will be normal or decreased in α-thalassemia and isolated iron deficiency anemia. There are several formulas to help in office screening, but they are also based on the assumption that the child is not iron deficient. Usually iron deficiency can be ruled out using free erythrocyte protoporphyrin, transferrin saturation, or ferritin as a screening test in children who have a hypochromic microcytic anemia. The least expensive test is a trial of iron and a repeated hemogram after a month. A lead level should be obtained if there is an index of suspicion for lead toxicity.

Problems can still arise: If both α- and β-thalassemia coexist, the changes in Hgb A_2 and F will not be apparent and, as noted above, there are instances of normal or elevated levels of Hgb A_2 and F in β-thalassemia trait. Family studies and, if warranted, DNA analysis can be used to make a definitive diagnosis.

THALASSEMIA INTERMEDIA

Children who are diagnosed with thalassemia intermedia have a homozygous or heterozygous β-globin mutation that causes a decrease in beta chain production, but not to the degree that chronic transfusion therapy is required. The phenotype can also occur in children who have a mutation that increases production of γ-globin, in children who have co-inherited α-thalassemia and β-thalassemia, and in other rarer mutations. Children who have thalassemia intermedia are able to maintain a hemoglobin of 7 g/dl or slightly higher with a greatly expanded erythron, and may manifest bony deformities, pathologic fractures, and growth retardation. Children who have thalassemia intermedia can also have delayed pubescence, exercise intolerance, leg ulcers, inflammatory arthritis, and extramedullary hematopoiesis causing spinal cord compression, a medical emergency requiring radiation therapy and transfusion. They can also have iron overload as a result of increased absorption of iron from the gastrointestinal tract and intermittent transfusion. They are at risk for the cardiac and endocrine complications of hemosiderosis, but usually at an older age than chronically transfused children. Chelation therapy is indicated for increasing ferritin and elevated liver iron.

Children who cannot maintain a hemoglobin between 6 and 7 g/dl should have an alternative diagnosis considered. If thalassemia is the cause of the anemia, transfusion and/or splenectomy should be considered. Frequently, adolescents and adults are unable to tolerate the degree of anemia that is seen in thalassemia intermedia. Hypersplenism, splenic pain, congestive heart failure, severe exercise intolerance, thrombocytopenia, and leukopenia should be considered indications for transfusion and splenectomy.

β-THALASSEMIA MAJOR

Thalassemia major was first described by a Detroit pediatrician, Thomas Cooley, in 1925. The clinical picture he described is prevalent today in countries without the necessary resources to provide patients with chronic transfusions and deferoxamine therapy. Children who have untreated thalassemia major have ineffective erythropoiesis, decreased red cell deformability, and enhanced clearance of defective red cells by macrophages. The result is a very hypermetabolic bone marrow with thrombocytosis, leukocytosis, and microcytic anemia in the young child prior to the enlargement of the spleen. At presentation they have almost 100% Hgb F (these cells have a longer life span as a result of a balanced globin ratio because γ-, rather than β-, globin is present in Hgb F). These children have little or no Hgb A_2 and a low reticulocyte count. The diagnosis can be made with certainty by demonstrating thalassemia trait in both parents, by globin biosynthetic ratios, or by beta gene screening. Beta gene screening identifies the most common and some uncommon mutations, but not all mutations. An electrophoresis showing only Hgb F, a complete blood count, and a characteristic peripheral smear will generally be diagnostic. In most states, these children will be discovered by state screening or occasionally by the obstetrician who makes a diagnosis of thalassemia trait in the mother and obtains a family history of thalassemia or anemia in both parents prior to the birth of the baby.

Children who have untreated thalassemia die in the first decade of life from anemia, septicemia, and pathologic fractures. When palliative transfusions are introduced, children live into their late teens, eventually succumbing to heart failure resulting from iron overload. With the introduction of frequent chronic transfusion therapy and the use of small pumps to deliver deferoxamine subcutaneously, children are now surviving into adulthood, adding to the complexity of the disease. The longevity of patients who are compliant with their deferoxamine therapy or who have received bone marrow transplantation is not known.

NEONATAL SCREENING FOR HEMOGLOBINOPATHIES

All individuals who are diagnosed with hemoglobin H require alpha gene screening to detect the possibility of Hgb H–Constant Spring.

The presence of Hgb F only on the newborn screening will be interpreted as β-thalassemia major. This diagnosis must be confirmed with parental electrophoresis and repeated testing of the infant at 3 to 6 months. Hemoglobin FA is not interpreted as β-thalassemia trait. This is a diagnosis made by the practitioner when microcytic anemia is seen during routine childhood screening and an investigation for thalassemia confirms the diagnosis.

Hemoglobin EF or Hgb FE will be presumed to be Hgb E–β-thalassemia until that diagnosis is investigated and confirmed, or ruled out by repeat electrophoresis and family studies. Hemoglobin E is the most common abnormal hemoglobin discovered in the state of California on newborn screening. It is common in Laos, Cambodia, and Thailand. Hemoglobin E results from a mutation in an exon (exon 1, codon 26: GAG to AAG) that creates an alternate splice site competing with the normal splice site. This results in abnormal hemoglobin production and mild thalassemia in the homozygous state. In the homozygous state, it produces a mild microcytic anemia with a hemoglobin usually above 10 g/dl. Electrophoresis reveals about 90% Hgb E with varying amounts of Hgb F. The heterozygote has a hemoglobin of about 12 g/dl with microcytosis and an electrophoretic pattern consistent with Hgb E plus Hgb A_2 of 20% to 30%. When combined with other more severe β-thalassemias, Hgb E–β-thalassemia can produce an anemia that is profound, requiring chronic transfusion therapy (a rare event compared to the high incidence of Hgb E and other β-thalassemias).

All children who have Hgb E and Hgb F on their state screen require scrutiny for emergence of a severe thalassemia syndrome. Individuals who have Hgb EE do not have a significant anemia and do not require special care except that they should *not* be treated with iron for anemia.

SUGGESTED READING

Hastings CA, Lubin BH. Blood. In: Rudolph AM, Kamei RK (eds), Rudolph's Fundamentals of Pediatrics, 2nd ed. Norwalk, CT: Appleton & Lange, 1998, pp 441–490.

Orkin SH, Nathan DG. The thalassemias. In: Nathan DG, Orkin SH (eds), Nathan and Oski's Hematology of Infancy and Childhood, 5th ed. Philadelphia: WB Saunders, 1998, pp 811–886.

TRANSFUSION THERAPY

BLOOD PRODUCTS

Transfusion of blood products continues to be an important and necessary part of therapy in children with hematologic or oncologic diagnoses. Many potential complications may arise, both infectious and noninfectious. With continued improvements in donor screening, and better testing techniques for infection, complications and infections are decreasing rapidly. However, as long as blood component therapy is derived from human blood donations, the risks will persist. These risks must be carefully considered in addition to the expected benefits each time a transfusion is contemplated. Informed consent should be obtained prior to every nonemergent transfusion.

Clerical errors and misidentification are major risks for transfusion and can result in serious consequences, including death. It is essential that all blood samples drawn for a type and cross-match be clearly labeled with the patient's identification. Before administration of the blood product, the order should be checked, patient identification reviewed (patient's identification band), and blood type verified.

Directed donation from first-degree relatives should be discouraged for patients who may be candidates for an allogeneic bone marrow transplant because of the possibility of antigen sensitization. If it cannot be avoided, the blood should be irradiated to prevent graft-versus-host disease (GVHD).

Donor selection criteria are designed to screen out potential donors with increased risk of infection with human immunodeficiency virus types 1 and 2, human T-lymphotropic virus types I and II, and hepatitis B and C, as well as other infectious pathogens. Despite rigorous screening and testing for these infections, the risk of transmitting these viruses is not totally eliminated. Pathogens known to be transmitted by transfusion include *Babesia* species, *Bartonella* species, *Borrelia* species, *Brucella* species, Colorado tick fever, *Leishmania* species, *Parvovirus,* plasmodia, rickettsia, *Toxoplasma* species, and certain trypanosomas.

RED BLOOD CELLS

Transfusion decisions are made on the basis of clinical context, not a number. Prior to transfusion, it is necessary to assess the mechanism responsible for anemia (bone marrow infiltration, ineffective erythropoiesis of chronic disease, occult or obvious blood loss, transfusion or drug-related suppression of normal hematopoiesis, nutritional deficiency); the severity of the signs and symptoms; and the likelihood of resumption of normal hematopoiesis.

One unit of packed red blood cells (PRBCs) is approximately 225 to 350 ml, with a hematocrit of approximately 55% to 65%. The majority of platelets and white blood cells (WBCs) have been removed during the processing. It is the product of choice to restore red cell mass and oxygen-carrying capacity. PRBCs need to be ABO and Rh(D) compatible.

Leukocyte filters remove more than 99.9% of the leukocytes, resulting in fewer febrile reactions and less alloimmunization. Washed PRBCs also result in a leukocyte-depleted unit while preserving 70% to 85% of the red cell mass; however, this is an expensive and usually unnecessary process. The primary indication for washing is to remove plasma. Greater than 85% of the leukocytes are removed, as well as 99% of the original plasma.

INDICATIONS FOR RED CELL TRANSFUSION
Packed Red Blood Cells

1. Infants less than 4 months old
   a. Venous hemoglobin level less than 13 g/dl in neonates less than 24 hours old
   b. Hemoglobin level less than 13 g/dl and severe pulmonary disease, cyanotic heart disease, or heart failure
   c. Acute blood loss of 10% or more of total blood volume
   d. Phlebotomy losses of 5% to 10% or more of the total blood volume
   e. Hemoglobin level less than 8 g/dl in stable newborn infants with clinical manifestations of anemia
2. Patients 4 months of age or older
   a. Significant preoperative or postoperative anemia: intraoperative blood loss of 10% to 15% or more of total blood volume, postoperative hemoglobin level less than 8 g/dl, and symptoms or signs of anemia
   b. Acute blood loss with hypovolemia unresponsive to crystalloid or colloid
3. Chronic congenital or acquired anemia without an expected satisfactory response to medical therapy and a hemoglobin level less than 8 g/dl with symptoms and/or signs of anemia
4. Chronic transfusions to suppress endogenous red cell production in patients with sickle cell disease or thalassemia syndromes

Whole Blood (Seldom Used)

1. Massive transfusion or acute blood loss (>1 blood volume in <24 hours), usually associated with trauma
2. Cardiovascular bypass surgery
3. Extracorporeal membrane oxygenation

SPECIAL REQUIREMENTS FOR PACKED RED BLOOD CELL TRANSFUSION
Sickle Cell Disease

Straight or exchange transfusion is often indicated for patients with stroke, acute chest syndrome, splenic sequestration, priapism, presurgical status, aplastic crises, and severe and frequent pain episodes (see Chapter 3).

The antigenic phenotype of the red cells (at least the ABO, Rh, Kell,

Duffy, Kidd, Lutheran, P, and MNS groups) should be determined in all patients older than 6 months of age. The record of the phenotype should be maintained in the blood bank.

All patients with a history of prior transfusion should be screened for the presence of alloantibodies. The high prevalence of alloimmunization in sickle cell disease most likely has several causes, but lack of phenotypic compatibility between the donor and recipient is a major factor. All patients should receive limited **phenotypically matched blood** (for antigens E, C, and Kell). Extensive phenotypic matching is recommended for patients who have developed antibodies.

Acute events may necessitate exchange transfusion to decrease the percentage of Hgb S and reverse sickling. Long-term management may require chronic transfusion therapy to suppress hematopoiesis and production of excess Hgb S. Erythrocytapheresis is now frequently performed rather than straight transfusion. Patients who are very anemic may benefit from a PRBC transfusion for acute pain or infection-related problems.

All blood should be screened for the presence of sickle hemoglobin, such as by solubility testing, and confirmed to be negative. This procedure eliminates blood with sickle cell trait, which would later confuse the measurement of Hgb S.

Prestorage **leukocyte depletion** of red cells is standard practice because of reduction in febrile reactions, platelet refractoriness, infections, and cytokine-induced complications. Washed red cells should be reserved for patients with a history of allergic reactions following prior transfusion.

Irradiated blood transfusions should be considered in patients likely to be candidates for bone marrow transplantation. These children should not receive blood from relatives.

Autologous blood transfusion should be avoided in sickle cell disease. Red cell substitutes are currently experimental and not indicated.

Oncology

Oncology patients are commonly anemic at diagnosis as a result of marrow involvement and treatment with myelosuppressive chemotherapy. The optimal hemoglobin level cannot be precisely defined and is dependent on the clinical situation. The following are specific guidelines for transfusion:

1. Stable, asymptomatic child recovering from treatment-induced anemia with hemoglobin less than 7 g/dl and a low reticulocyte count
2. Symptomatic anemia and hemoglobin less than 10 g/dl
3. Hemoglobin less than 8 g/dl in a patient beginning an induction or intensification course of chemotherapy, especially acute myelogenous leukemia (AML) patients
4. Acute blood loss of greater than 10% of total blood volume or ongoing loss and a hemoglobin of less than 8 g/dl in a child unable to produce red cells
5. Hemoglobin less than 7 g/dl prior to general anesthesia

6. Children receiving radiation therapy, who may require a hemoglobin level of 10 g/dl or greater

DOSAGE

In a severely anemic child without hypovolemia, small incremental transfusions with PRBCs are indicated. Each 3 to 5 ml/kg should be given over 4 hours until the desired hemoglobin is achieved. Furosemide may be needed midtransfusion to prevent fluid overload. The blood bank should be notified of the need for repeated small aliquot transfusions, so as to partition the unit(s) and minimize donor exposures for the patient.

In general, transfuse to a hemoglobin of 10 to 13 g/dl, depending on the patient's diagnosis and clinical status and the size of the units. Transfusing 10 ml/kg will increase the hemoglobin by approximately 3 g/dl. Round off to the nearest unit to avoid wasting a small quantity and avoid exposure of the patient to a second donor for a small quantity. *For patients with sickle cell disease, be careful not to transfuse over 12 g/dl because of the risk of hyperviscosity and increased risk of central nervous system events.* For oncology patients, transfusion to a "normal" hemoglobin is acceptable and warranted as long as excess donor exposure is avoided.

For stable patients with hemoglobins over 5 g/dl, the transfusion can be given over 2 to 4 hours (units cannot be given over longer periods of time unless partitioned by the blood bank because of expiration times).

A hemoglobin level should be checked 2 to 4 hours after completion of the transfusion to allow time for equilibration.

Exchange transfusion, or **erythrocytapheresis,** may be indicated in the severely anemic patient with congestive heart failure, acute sickle cell events, hyperleukocytosis, or hyperbilirubinemia, or in an anemic patient treated with severe fluid restriction (increased intracranial pressure). In sickle cell disease, exchange transfusion quickly reduces the concentration of sickle cells without increasing the hematocrit or whole blood viscosity. Red cell exchange transfusion has the potential to reduce the iron accumulation because an equal volume of red cells are removed as the Hgb A–containing cells are infused. Automated erythrocytapheresis can be done rapidly and safely in most situations. Limitations of this technique include increased red cell utilization, venous access, and increased cost. Important considerations include the following:

1. A single volume exchange is an exchange of 80 ml/kg.
2. Reconstitute PRBCs in 5% albumin or normal saline to a hemoglobin of 10 g/dl for sickle cell patients (fresh frozen plasma [FFP] is not necessary). Reconstitute to a hemoglobin of 10 to 12 g/dl for patients with a desired higher ending hemoglobin.
3. Exchange equal aliquots, unless a higher or lower ending hemoglobin is desired, in all cases in which exchange transfusion is used be certain that the final hemoglobin does not exceed 10 to 12 g/dl to avoid the problems of hyperviscosity in children with sickle cell

disease. The hemoglobin in children with hyperleukocytosis should not exceed 8 to 10 g/dl. Careful monitoring of the level of hemoglobin and the percentage of Hgb A and Hgb S (in sickle cell disease) or WBCs (in hyperleukocytosis) is necessary to be certain that the goals of transfusion have been met.

4. Patients receiving large quantities of blood may develop hypocalcemia because of the preparation method, which involves anticoagulation with calcium chelation. Calcium gluconate may need to be given during an exchange transfusion or massive transfusion with whole blood or PRBCs.

PLATELETS

Platelet transfusions are indicated for thrombocytopenic patients with bleeding resulting from severely decreased platelet production or for patients with bleeding and functionally abnormal platelets. They are not indicated for those patients with rapid destruction (immune thrombocytopenic purpura [ITP]) unless there is a life-threatening hemorrhage. They may be useful in the bleeding patient with rapid consumption (disseminated intravascular coagulation [DIC]) or dilutional thrombocytopenia (massive transfusion or exchange). They are frequently needed in the patient receiving chemotherapy or who is thrombocytopenic secondary to a marrow infiltrative process.

INDICATIONS
Premature or Sick Infants
1. Stable infant with platelet count less than 50×10^9/L
2. Distressed infant with platelet count less than 100×10^9/L

Children
1. Platelet count less than 10×10^9/L, or higher if febrile, infected, or bleeding
2. Platelet count less than 50×10^9/L with an anticipated invasive procedure
   a. Lumbar puncture
   b. Extracorporeal membrane oxygenation or cardiovascular bypass
   c. Qualitative platelet defect
   d. Surgery (central line replacement)

Oncology
1. Nonbleeding patient with platelet count less than 10×10^9/L
2. Induction chemotherapy: acute lymphocytic leukemia in patient with platelet count less than 10 to 15×10^9/L; AML patient with platelet count less than 20×10^9/L
3. Children with brain tumors, who should have their platelet count maintained at 30×10^9/L or greater
4. Lumbar puncture with platelet count less than 30 to 50×10^9/L

5. Bleeding patient with normal coagulation studies, platelet count less than 50×10^9/L
6. Patient requiring a surgical procedure, with platelet count less than 100×10^9/L
7. Intramuscular injection with platelet count less than 20×10^9/L

DOSAGE

One unit of random platelets per 10 kg will increase the platelet count by 40 to 50×10^9/L if there is no active consumptive process (fever, ITP, sepsis, alloimmunization, DIC) or sequestration. The platelet count should be checked 1 to 2 hours after infusion to identify refractory patients. A patient is refractory if, 1 hour after transfusion, the platelet increment is less than 5 to 10×10^9/L per unit transfused for two separate transfusions.

A patient may have platelet refractoriness secondary to alloantibodies (immune mediated). Nonimmune causes of platelet refractoriness are common and include splenomegaly, fever, infection, DIC, and use of amphotericin.

For refractory patients, a trial of cross-matched platelets should be given. Other possibilities for treatment should this fail include leukocyte-depleted, human lymphocyte antigen (HLA)-matched platelets, intravenous immune globulin with HLA-matched platelets, or massive transfusion with random donor platelets (to overwhelm the antibody concentration).

Pheresis platelets are harvested from a single donor and generally contain greater than 30×10^9/L platelets, which equals approximately 6 to 8 units of random platelets. The volume is usually 250 to 300 ml. This is the preferable platelet preparation to use. Single-donor apheresed platelets are indicated for patients who are frequently transfused or need multiple units (i.e., most patients) so as to decrease donor exposure and the inherent risks. The units can be split for more efficient use. ABO-compatible platelets are recommended, but ABO-incompatible units may be used if not grossly contaminated by red blood cells (RBCs).

GRANULOCYTES

Granulocytes are used for supportive treatment of selected patients with neutropenia (absolute neutrophil count [ANC] $<100/\mu$l) and infection documented by persistent positive culture with gram-negative organisms or fungus, despite appropriate therapy. Granulocytes migrate toward, phagocytize, and kill bacteria. When a patient is given a granulocyte transfusion, the cells migrate to the foci of infection, though there is rarely a measurable increase in the peripheral granulocyte count. This is likely because of sequestration or prior immunization to leukocyte antigens or a consumptive process associated with infection. In patients whose donors have been primed with granulocyte colony-stimulating factor and steroids prior to donation, transient elevation of peripheral counts may be seen in the recipients. Side effects of granulocyte transfusions include the risk of cytomegalovirus (CMV) infection, GVHD, respiratory distress with pulmonary infiltrates, alloimmunization, and hemolytic reactions.

A bag or unit of granulocytes contains a large number of granulocytes (1.0×10^{10} cells) in addition to other leukocytes, platelets, and 20 to 50 ml of RBCs. Donors may be premedicated with steroids to increase the circulating pool of granulocytes. A unit of granulocytes is from a single donor. The granulocytes are resuspended in approximately 200 to 300 ml of anticoagulated plasma. Donors are ABO/Rh compatible, HLA matched, and anti-neutrophil antibody negative. Granulocytes should be from CMV-negative donors and irradiated because the recipients are immune compromised. The circulating half-life of granulocytes is 6 to 10 hours.

INDICATIONS

1. Neonatal bacterial sepsis
2. Bacterial (or fungal) sepsis, culture positive or deep seated, unresponsive to antimicrobial treatment, ANC less than $100/\mu l$ or qualitative neutrophil defect, neutrophil count not expected to increase over $500/\mu l$ for several days

DOSAGE

A unit of granulocytes should be administered at 150 ml/m^2/hour as soon as possible after collection and be separated as far in time as possible from amphotericin infusions. Do not administer with a leukocyte-depleting filter. Units are given daily until the ANC is above $100/\mu l$ and the infection is resolving.

PLASMA

FFP is a source of plasma proteins, including nonlabile clotting factors such as fibrinogen. It is used for the treatment of stable clotting factor deficiencies in which no concentrate is available (*not* for factor VIII or IX). Serum refers to plasma that is devoid of coagulation proteins. By definition, each milliliter of undiluted plasma contains 1 international unit (IU) of each coagulation factor.

Plasma consists of the anticoagulated clear portion of blood separated by centrifugation. FFP is plasma that has been separated and frozen within 6 hours of collection. A bag of FFP contains 200 units of factor VIII. FFP should not be used when the coagulopathy can be corrected more effectively with specific treatment such as vitamin K, cryoprecipitate, or factor concentrate. Cryoprecipitate is prepared by thawing FFP and recovering the cold precipitate. Each bag contains more than 80 units of factor VIII coagulant and more than 150 mg fibrinogen in approximately 15 ml of plasma. It is a good source of factors VIII, XIII, fibrinogen, and von Willebrand factor. Bags must usually be pooled to achieve an adequate dose. Plasma must be ABO compatible with the recipient's red cells; Rh does not need to be considered. Compatibility tests are not necessary for cryoprecipitate. Antibodies in the plasma may react with the recipient's RBCs, and a Coombs' test can reflect this.

INDICATIONS
Fresh Frozen Plasma
1. Bleeding or invasive procedure with documented clotting factor deficiency and appropriate factor not available
2. Treatment of antithrombin III (AT III), protein C or S deficiency, or factor XI deficiency (hemophilia C)
3. Bleeding during massive transfusion, not from thrombocytopenia

Cryoprecipitate
1. Bleeding or invasive procedure with factor VIII deficiency or von Willebrand disease and factor concentrate not available
2. Bleeding or invasive procedure with hypofibrinogenemia or factor XIII deficiency
3. Supportive treatment for DIC (after controlling for etiologic factors)
4. Hypofibrinogenemia secondary to asparaginase therapy in oncology patients (treat for fibrinogen less than 40 to 50 mg/dl; if patient is symptomatic, treat for fibrinogen less than 100 mg/dl)

DOSAGE
The usual dosage of FFP is 10 to 15 ml/kg. The usual dosage for cryoprecipitate is 1 U/6 kg. Obtain a fibrinogen level at 30 minutes postinfusion. For hypofibrinogenemia with coagulopathy, the goal is to maintain fibrinogen greater than 100 mg/dl. Specific factor or coagulation protein levels need to be determined, in addition to assessing clinical status, to decide on frequency of transfusion.

ANTITHROMBIN III
AT III concentrate is available for use in patients with inherited or acquired AT III deficiency (sepsis, thrombosis, medication). It may also be needed in patients receiving heparin therapy who have a low AT III level. Refer to package insert for dosing.

PREPARATION OF BLOOD PRODUCTS

IRRADIATION
Blood components may be irradiated to prevent GVHD by preventing the proliferation of T lymphocytes. Blood components can receive 2500 cGy without affecting the therapeutic dose and benefit of the blood product.

Irradiated blood is indicated for patients at risk for GVHD from transfusion. These patients include neonates and immune-compromised patients (underlying malignancy, receiving chemotherapy, and marrow or stem cell transplant recipient). Red cells, platelets, and granulocytes can be irradiated. Irradiation induces red cell membrane damage, resulting in an elevated plasma potassium. Removal of residual supernatant prior to transfusion may reduce the risks associated with an elevated potassium level.

CYTOMEGALOVIRUS TESTING

Seronegative blood is selected by performing testing for antibodies to CMV. Because CMV is associated with cellular blood components, FFP, cryoprecipitate, and other plasma-derived blood components do not require special testing. Transfusion of CMV-negative blood products is indicated for immune-suppressed patients (neonates and patients with malignancies likely to receive a bone marrow transplant) who are CMV negative.

LEUKOCYTE DEPLETION

Leukocyte-reduced blood is prepared by filtering blood with special filters that remove white cells by sieving and adherence mechanisms. Filtration is preferably done at the time of collection for quality control testing, but may also be done at the bedside. Leukocyte filtration is done on whole blood, RBCs, and platelets. Leukocyte-reduced components are indicated for immune-suppressed individuals to remove leukocytes potentially harboring CMV; prevent recurrent febrile, nonhemolytic transfusion reactions; and reduce the incidence of HLA alloimmunization.

SUGGESTED READING

American Association of Blood Banks. Administration of blood products. In: Technical Manual, 13th ed. Bethesda, MD: American Association of Blood Banks, 1999.

American Association of Blood Banks, America's Blood Centers, and the American Red Cross. Circular of Information for the Use of Human Blood and Blood Components. Bethesda, MD: American Association of Blood Banks, 2000.

Barnard DR, Feusner JH, Wolff LJ. Blood component therapy. In: Ablin AR (ed), Supportive Care of Children with Cancer, 2nd ed. Baltimore: The Johns Hopkins University Press, 1997, pp 37–46.

Reed W, Vichinsky EP. Transfusion therapy: a coming-of-age treatment for patients with sickle cell disease. J Pediatr Hematol Oncol 23:197–202, 2001.

TRANSFUSION REACTIONS

Approximately 4% of transfusions are associated with some form of adverse reaction, the majority being febrile nonhemolytic or urticarial reactions and a few being delayed hemolytic reactions. Children rarely have a febrile reaction with an initial transfusion unless they are immunoglobulin A (IgA) deficient. Life-threatening transfusion reactions are nearly always due to a clerical error when a unit is given to the wrong patient (i.e., ABO incompatible). For all transfusion reactions, a bedside check of all labels, forms, and patient identification should be done, in addition to notifying the blood bank. A postreaction blood sample (for typing and culture) from the patient should be sent with the implicated blood component.

ALLERGIC REACTIONS

Allergic reactions usually are manifested by urticaria, but may also induce wheezing or angioedematous reactions. These reactions may occur with the first transfusion.

If the reaction is localized, stop the transfusion and administer an antihistamine. Patients with repeated urticarial reactions should receive premedication with an antihistamine or corticosteroid and may need washed red cells with subsequent transfusions. If the reaction is mild and resolving with an antihistamine, the transfusion may be completed. In severe cases, corticosteroids or epinephrine may be needed to treat the reaction, and the transfusion should be discontinued altogether.

Anaphylactoid reactions are a rare but dangerous complication requiring immediate treatment with corticosteroids and epinephrine. These reactions may be clinically manifested by severe dyspnea, pulmonary and/or laryngeal edema, or bronchospasm/laryngospasm. The majority of these reactions have been reported in IgA-deficient patients who have IgA antibodies. Such patients may not have received prior transfusions and may develop symptoms after infusion of a very small amount of IgA-containing plasma.

Transfusion-related acute lung injury occurs when acutely increased permeability of the pulmonary microcirculation causes massive leakage of fluid and protein into the alveolar spaces and interstitium. This complication is rapid in onset, usually within 6 hours of transfusion. Granulocyte antibodies in the donor or recipient have been implicated, yet the mechanism of action is unclear. Treatment consists of aggressive respiratory support.

FEBRILE NONHEMOLYTIC REACTIONS

Fever, chills, or diaphoresis during a transfusion are almost always due to a reaction between antibodies in the host and leukocyte or plasma protein alloantigens in the blood product. These symptoms may also be cytokine mediated.

Such a reaction requires formation of antibodies and occurs exclusively in patients with a prior history of transfusion or pregnancy.

Chronically transfused patients should always receive leukocyte-depleted blood products to avoid febrile reactions to white blood cells or plasma. Washed packed red blood cells (PRBCs) or IgA-deficient plasma may be needed for further transfusions.

Treatment consists of immediately stopping the transfusion, evaluating the patient (vital signs, exam, blood cultures), treating the patient's symptoms (acetaminophen), and evaluating the blood product (culture, re-cross-match). Table 6–1 lists the drugs used in the treatment of nonhemolytic transfusion reactions.

TABLE 6–1
DRUGS USED IN THE TREATMENT OF NONHEMOLYTIC TRANSFUSION REACTIONS

Diphenhydramine	*Use:* Treating pruritus and rash (hives)
	Dose: 12.5–50 mg IV over 10–20 minutes (1 mg/kg/dose, maximum dose 50 mg)
Epinephrine	*Use:* Severe reactions characterized by bronchospasm, hypotension, shock
(1:1000 aqueous) (1 mg/ml)	*Dose:* 0.01 ml/kg SQ (Single dose maximum 1 mg). Repeat q15min × 3–4 doses as needed. For patients in shock not responding to epinephrine, an initial fluid bolus treatment should be given. As in patients with shock from other causes, fluids, vasopressors, airway protection, oxygenation, etc., should also be used.
Epinephrine (Sus-Phrine) (1:200 aqueous) (1.5 mg/0.3 ml)	*Use:* Following stabilization with epinephrine. *Dose:* 0.005 ml/kg SQ (maximum single dose 0.15 ml) Repeat q8–12h PRN.
Fluids	For hypotensive patients, a bolus of 20 ml/kg of normal saline should be administered simultaneously with epinephrine and steroids.
Narcotics	*Use:* Specific and effective treatment for rigors *Dose:* 0.1 mg/kg morphine IV (maximum dose 10 mg)
Acetaminophen	*Use:* To prevent or reverse temperature elevations in mild to moderate febrile reactions *Dose:* 10–15 mg/kg PO (maximum dose 800 mg)
Steroids	*Use:* In moderate to severe reactions; may occasionally be required in severe urticaria. Indicated in all reactions characterized by fever, shaking, chills, diaphoresis, or pallor. *Dose:* 1–2 mg/kg of methylprednisolone (or equivalent dose of dexamethasone/hydrocortisone) IV push.

Adapted from Kevy SV, Gorlin JB. Red cell transfusion. In: Nathan DG, Orkin SH (eds), Nathan and Oski's Hematology of Infancy and Childhood, 5th ed. Philadelphia: WB Saunders, 1998, pp 1784–1801.

ACUTE HEMOLYTIC TRANSFUSION REACTIONS

Hemolytic transfusion reactions result in the immunologic destruction of transfused red cells, nearly always as a result of incompatibility of antigen on the transfused cells with antibody in the recipient's circulation. The most common cause of severe reactions is transfusion of ABO-incompatible blood, resulting from clerical or identification errors.

Acute hemolytic reactions are characterized by fever, chills, urticaria, dyspnea, chest pain, abdominal or lower back pain, tachycardia, hypertension or hypotension, renal failure, jaundice, and shock.

Laboratory evaluation includes complete blood count, coagulation studies, urinalysis, and a direct Coombs' test. Findings may include anemia, disseminated intravascular coagulation, hemoglobinemia, hemoglobinuria, and a positive Coombs' test. Free plasma hemoglobin may rise rapidly, followed by an elevation of serum bilirubin.

Treatment is *immediate cessation of transfusion* and administration of *fluids, steroids, mannitol,* and *pressors* as needed to maintain cardiovascular stability and maintain urine flow. **Caution:** sudden pain, jaundice, and anemia in sickle cell patients may be mistaken for an acute pain event.

DELAYED TRANSFUSION REACTIONS

Occasionally, patients receiving compatible red cells may experience symptoms of a hemolytic reaction 2 to 14 days later. These patients have been sensitized to one or more "minor" blood group antigens during a prior transfusion. The titers may fall to undetectable levels between transfusions. During re-exposure, an anamnestic response occurs and, when sufficient antibody is produced, clinical hemolysis occurs. These transfusions can result in profound anemia, though usually milder than that with ABO incompatibility.

Signs of a delayed transfusion reaction may include unexplained fever, development of a positive direct Coombs' test, and anemia. Hyperbilirubinemia and hemoglobinuria are uncommon. Elevated lactate dehydrogenase or bilirubin may be noted. New red cell antibodies may be identified in the patient. The direct Coombs' test may be negative if all the transfused cells already have hemolyzed.

Most delayed transfusion reactions have a benign course and require no therapeutic intervention.

ALLOIMMUNIZATION

Alloimmunization may occur unpredictably following transfusion of red cells, platelets, plasma, or white cells. Primary immunization does not usually cause any symptoms or physiologic changes. However, if subsequent exposure to the relative antigens occurs with further transfusion, there may be accelerated removal of cellular elements from the circulation, possibly associated with systemic symptoms.

6

ALLOIMMUNIZATION

GRAFT-VERSUS-HOST DISEASE

Graft-versus-host disease (GVHD) is a rare but dangerous complication that occurs when viable T lymphocytes from the transfused component engraft in the recipient and react against tissue antigens. Severely immune-compromised recipients are at greatest risk (fetuses, neonates, severe immunodeficiency, and recipients of bone marrow or stem cell transplants), though GVHD has been reported in immunologically normal recipients heterozygous for a tissue antigen haplotype for which the donor is homozygous. This most likely occurs when the donor is a blood relative or has been selected for human lymphocyte antigen compatibility. Leukocyte depletion does reduce T lymphocytes, though sufficient numbers are left behind to still cause GVHD. Irradiation of the blood component is the only approved means of preventing GVHD by rendering T lymphocytes incapable of proliferation.

BACTERIAL CONTAMINATION

Bacterial contamination rarely occurs, but can cause acute, severe, life-threatening hypotension and circulatory collapse. Severe chills or cardiovascular compromise during or immediately after transfusion suggest the possibility of bacterial contamination and/or endotoxin reaction. Gram-positive and gram-negative organisms can cause septic shock. The transfusion should be discontinued immediately and aggressive therapy initiated with broad-spectrum antibiotics and vasopressors as needed. Prompt investigation should include blood cultures (including Gram's stain) from the patient, the blood component, and the administration set.

SUGGESTED READING

American Association of Blood Banks, America's Blood Centers, and the American Red Cross. Circular of Information for the Use of Human Blood and Blood Components. Bethesda, MD: American Association of Blood Banks 2000.

Kevy SV, Gorlin JB. Red cell transfusion. In: Nathan DG, Orkin SH (eds), Nathan and Oski's Hematology of Infancy and Childhood, 5th ed. Philadelphia: WB Saunders, 1998, pp 1784–1801.

CHELATION THERAPY

7

CHELATION FOR TRANSFUSIONAL IRON OVERLOAD

Iron overload may occur in any patient receiving intermittent transfusions for acute illness (e.g., sickle cell disease) or chronic transfusion therapy (thalassemia, sickle cell disease, red cell aplasia, bone marrow failure syndromes), or who has received an intensive period of frequent transfusions (myelosuppressive chemotherapy/radiation for treatment of malignancy). Each unit of blood contains approximately 250 mg of elemental iron. Patients receiving frequent transfusion should be monitored for evidence of iron accumulation.

DIAGNOSIS OF IRON OVERLOAD

There is no simple test for determining iron overload. Serial serum ferritin levels are helpful in determining iron stores, but unreliable because ferritin is an acute-phase reactant and levels are markedly altered by liver disease, inflammation, and vitamin C stores. Liver biopsy is the most accurate test for iron overload and is safe if performed by an experienced physician. Magnetic resonance imaging and computed tomography have been used to noninvasively measure organ iron content, but their clinical use is unproven. The super-conducting quantum interference device (SQUID) is accepted as a noninvasive method to quantitate liver iron, but its limited availability does not allow for routine use.

The best indicator for chelation is elevated liver iron stores. Some programs recommend liver biopsies at the initiation of chelation, and then every 2 years. Chelation therapy should begin when the liver iron is 7 mg/g dry weight. Alternatively, cumulative transfusions of 120 ml or more of packed red cells/kg/year can be used. Ferritin levels of above 1000 ng/ml in the steady state are helpful, but the risk of under- or overtreatment exists with this measure alone. All patients receiving chelation therapy should have frequent monitoring of iron stores and organ toxicity, in addition to ongoing education and support.

CHELATION THERAPY

The **goal** of chelation therapy is to maintain the total body iron load in a near-normal range. The most commonly used drug for iron chelation is deferoxamine. Deferoxamine was isolated from *Streptomyces pilosus* in the 1960s. It is used subcutaneously and intravenously to chelate iron in all children who have hemosiderosis secondary to chronic transfusions. Other chelators are undergoing safety and efficacy studies, and are not recommended at this time.

Deferoxamine is not without **side effects**. The most common is ototoxicity, manifested by tinnitus and a transient hearing loss. Other side effects include ophthalmologic effects (decreased night vision), allergic reactions, growth failure, unusual infections, and pulmonary hypersensitivity. Despite these potential problems, deferoxamine is generally considered a safe medication. It should not be given in pregnancy and renal disease. An expected acute reaction with a SQ injection is a localized erythematous rash. Hydrocortisone can be mixed with deferoxamine to decrease this reaction. A common occurrence is irritation at the site of administration; this can be decreased by diluting the deferoxamine. Patients receiving deferoxamine are monitored closely for acute and late effects of this chelator, in addition to the effects of iron overload.

The most common problem encountered with the administration of deferoxamine is **compliance**. This chelator does remove iron, but only if used. Adolescent patients and some parents frequently miss doses or do not give the drug at all. A rising or unchanging ferritin level is frequently a sign of noncompliance, not inadequate dosage.

Deferoxamine is given **subcutaneously** at a dose of 20 to 50 mg/kg (usual starting dose is 25 mg/kg) over 8 to 10 hours, 3 to 5 nights per week. Ascorbic acid (vitamin C), 100 mg, will increase the excretion of iron and is given with the deferoxamine. If there is severe hemosiderosis, deferoxamine is given IV at a dose of 100 mg/kg over 12 hours. It is desirable to keep the ferritin level below 2000 ng/ml; if the ferritin level is above 4000 ng/ml, hospital admission should be considered for high-dose deferoxamine therapy. New methods of delivery are being studied.

Deferoxamine is not administered when an infection is present. By mobilizing free iron, it promotes bacterial growth, in particular that of *Yersinia enterocolitica*. When a patient receiving deferoxamine is febrile, chelation should be stopped until blood cultures are shown to be negative. Broad-spectrum coverage with antibiotics should include the possibility of this unusual organism.

CHELATION FOR ACUTE LEAD TOXICITY

Lead poisoning is an environmental disease the management of which has undergone a major evolution in the past few decades. Recognition of the devastating neurologic effects of high lead levels and knowledge of the causes have led to universal efforts to decrease environmental lead contamination, with a resultant decrease in measured blood lead levels in children over the past 2 to 3 decades. Sources of lead have included gasoline additives, food can soldering, lead-based paints, ceramic glazes, drinking water systems (lead pipes), and folk remedies. The use of these products has been markedly reduced as a result of federal guidelines and the development of cost-effective alternatives. Lead is at extremely low levels in gasoline and paint and has been eliminated altogether from food can soldering. Housing built prior to 1960 is still likely to have been painted with high-content lead-based paint, and, because lead isotopes are very stable, environmental exposure presents an ongoing risk. High-risk populations have a greater likelihood of living in older housing that has not had lead abatement. Risk factors for excessive lead exposure include poverty, age younger than 6 years, African-American ethnicity, and dwelling in the city.

Lead may enter the body through direct ingestion or inhalation, or via skin absorption. The most common pathway among young children is through the mouth. Pica enhances this behavior. Toddlers in particular are at risk, with normal behavior being to put objects and toys in the mouth and chew on unusual surfaces (window sills). Lead absorption is enhanced in the presence of other dietary mineral deficiencies, such as calcium and iron, as a result of competitive biochemical pathways.

CLINICAL EFFECTS OF LEAD

Lead entering the intravascular space rapidly attaches to the red blood cell, with minimal amounts (3%) detected in the plasma. The half-life in the blood is approximately 21 to 30 days. Excretion is primarily through the kidneys, with small amounts deposited in the hair, nails, and bile. The lead that remains in the body accumulates mostly in the bone (65% to 90%). Lead can enter any cell, and toxicity may occur in any tissue or organ. Classically, in severe lead intoxication, gastrointestinal and central nervous system toxicities are most clinically apparent. Gastrointestinal symptoms include anorexia, nausea, vomiting, abdominal pain, and constipation. The blood lead level is typically 50 μg/dl or greater when these symptoms are present. Lead poisoning was a lethal disease in the United States decades ago, primarily because of its neurotoxic effects. At levels above 100 μg/dl, children may show evidence of encephalopathy, including a marked change in mentation or activity, ataxia, seizures, and coma. Increased intracranial pressure may be present on examination. These effects are usually permanent, with long-term sequelae of retardation, palsies, and growth failure.

Most children who have elevated blood lead levels have subclinical disease. Fewer than 5% of children present with overt symptoms of lead toxicity. An elevated blood lead level, suggesting excessive environmental exposure, is defined as 10 μg/dl. Many studies have shown associations between blood lead levels and impaired neurocognitive function. These results have provided the primary impetus for current public health efforts.

PREVENTION AND TREATMENT

Prevention and treatment of lead toxicity is a major public health concern at this time, and efforts for screening have primarily focused on high-risk populations. All children should have a screen of potential environmental exposures by their health caregivers starting at 1 year of age, and repeated when the child is mobile and attains hand-to-mouth behavior. The Centers for Disease Control (CDC) and American Academy of Pediatrics (AAP) recommend lead blood sampling for children identified to be at high risk (living in housing built prior to 1960, indigent, urban, minority children). If the screening test confirms an elevated blood lead level, specific management guidelines have been developed by the CDC and AAP to assist with therapy.

Blood lead levels measure the blood concentration at a given point in time and may not be able to accurately predict bone stores. Bone lead content may be assessed noninvasively using a novel radiographic technique called x-ray fluorescence. Measurement of the heme precursor, free erythrocyte protoporphyrin (FEP), may also provide a useful clue about the duration of exposure and the degree of lead accumulation. Excessively high FEP levels classically are seen with severe lead toxicity. Other causes of elevated FEP levels include iron deficiency, inflammatory disorders, elevated bilirubin, and, rarely, porphyria.

The primary aims of treatment are prevention of future lead exposure and absorption and enhancement of excretion. The steps to accomplish these goals include the following:

1. Assess the environment to eliminate the sources or remove the child from the contaminated environment
2. Modify the child's behavior to decrease hand-to-mouth activity
3. Ensure adequate nutrition, especially minerals, to limit lead absorption
4. Administer medications (chelators) in children with very high lead levels to increase lead excretion

The vast majority of children with elevated lead levels are not candidates for chelation therapy with currently available drugs. Children with low levels (between 10 and 25 μg/dl) are asymptomatic and unlikely to have significant increase in lead excretion with chelation. These children benefit primarily from decreased exposure. Venous blood samples should be used to assess blood lead levels. Capillary samples may give falsely low results.

LEAD CHELATION GUIDELINES (AAP)

1. Chelation treatment is not indicated in patients with blood lead levels of *less than 25 μg/dl*, although environmental intervention should occur.
2. Patients with blood lead levels *between 25 and 44 μg/dl* need aggressive environmental intervention but should not routinely receive chelation therapy. If blood lead levels persist in this range despite appropriate intervention, chelation with oral succimer has been suggested; however, a recent study showed little efficacy in reducing blood lead levels and impacting neurocognitive outcomes.
3. Patients with blood lead levels *between 45 and 70 μg/dl* should receive chelation therapy.
   a. A plain radiograph of the abdomen should be obtained to assess for enteral lead; if present, bowel decontamination may be considered.
   b. In the absence of CNS symptoms, patients should receive succimer 30 mg/kg/day for 5 days, followed by 20 mg/kg/day for 14 days.
   c. Children may need to be hospitalized initially to monitor for adverse effects, institute environmental abatement, and ensure compliance.

d. An alternative regimen is calcium disodium edetate (CaNa$_2$EDTA) 25 mg/kg/day for 5 days, IV infusion (continuous or intermittent); this regimen requires inpatient administration.

4. Patients with blood lead levels *greater than 70 µg/dl* or with clinical symptoms suggesting central nervous system toxicity require inpatient chelation therapy using the most efficacious parenteral agents available.

  a. Therapy is initiated with dimercaprol (BAL) 25 mg/kg/day IM, divided q4h; after the second dose of BAL, immediately follow with CaNa$_2$EDTA 50 mg/kg/day continuous IV for 3 to 5 days.

  b. Adequate hydration needs to be maintained to ensure renal excretion.

  c. After this initial treatment, subsequent courses may be BAL and CaNa$_2$EDTA or CaNa$_2$EDTA alone.

After chelation therapy, a period of re-equilibration of 10 to 14 days should be allowed, and another blood lead concentration obtained. Subsequent treatments should be based on these levels, using the criteria given above. Ongoing efforts should be made to prevent exposure in the child's environment and assure adequate nutrition. Family members and siblings should be screened as well.

SUGGESTED READING

Andrews NC, Bridges KR. Disorders of iron metabolism and sideroblastic anemia. In: Nathan DG, Orkin SH (eds), Nathan and Oski's Hematology of Infancy and Childhood, 5th ed. Philadelphia: WB Saunders, 1998, pp 423–462.

Committee on Drugs, American Academy of Pediatrics. Treatment guidelines for lead exposure in children. Pediatrics 96:155–160, 1995.

Markowitz M. Lead poisoning. Pediatr Rev 21:327–335, 2000.

Rogan WJ, Dietrich KN, Ware JH, et al. The effect of chelation therapy with succimer on neuropsychological development in children exposed to lead. N Engl J Med 344: 1421–1426, 2001.

THE CHILD WITH A BLEEDING DISORDER

INITIAL EVALUATION

Hemostasis requires a coordinated interaction between platelets, vascular endothelial cells, and plasma clotting factors. The sequence of hemostatic mechanisms can be divided into two parts: primary and secondary plugs. The primary hemostatic plug involves a platelet plug forming at the initial site of injury. The common clinical disorders that are associated with abnormalities of primary hemostasis are vascular abnormalities, qualitative abnormalities of the platelets, quantitative abnormalities of the platelets, and von Willebrand disease. An aberration in primary hemostasis is characterized by bleeding of the mucous membranes, epistaxis, and superficial ecchymoses. Typical manifestations are prolonged oozing from minor wounds or abrasions and abnormal intraoperative bleeding. The secondary hemostatic plug involves the various plasma procoagulant proteins forming a fibrin clot. An aberration in this system is characterized by bleeding from large vessels with subcutaneous, palpable hematomas, hemarthroses, or intramuscular hematomas. The hemophilias are examples of disorders in this category.

HISTORY

Assessment of the child with a suspected or known bleeding diathesis begins with a complete history. A summary of important points in the history of the child with a bleeding disorder is presented in Table 8–1. The nature of the bleeding should be explored, with particular attention to location, duration, frequency, and the measures necessary to stop it. Obtaining a previous history of bleeding associated with trauma or surgery, dental extraction, circumcision, appendectomy, tonsillectomy, and the like is also important. Inquiry should be made into a history of rash (petechial) or arthritis with hemarthrosis, and of blood transfusion. The first episode of bleeding should be documented, and a careful history of bruising during the toddler age is important. In females, the duration and severity of menstrual bleeding should be documented, as should excessive bleeding following childbirth in family members.

A family history and pedigree are crucial because many bleeding disorders are hereditary. The history should also address the use of over-the-counter and prescription drugs that can induce bleeding. The most common offenders are aspirin, ibuprofen, and naproxen. It is important to ask the patient specifically about the use of medications for colds, sinus trouble, muscle aches, or headaches, which may contain these medications. Some antibiotics, penicillin in particular, can affect platelet function or be associated with specific inhibitors of clotting. Anticonvulsants can cause thrombocytopenia, and procainamide has been associated with an acquired lupus anticoagulant.

TABLE 8–1

OBTAINING A BLEEDING HISTORY

MEDICAL HISTORY	FAMILY HISTORY
Spontaneous bleeding	Known bleeding diathesis
Age of onset	Excessive hemorrhage following
Bruising, petechiae (location)	childbirth; menorrhagia
Joint bleeding; muscle bleeding	Blood transfusions
Mucous membrane bleeding (epistaxis)	Gender of affected members
Menorrhagia	Family tree
Induced bleeding	
Injuries	
Duration of bleeding; nature of injuries	
What it takes to stop the bleeding	
Wound healing	
History of transfusions	
Surgical procedures	
Circumcision	
Tonsillectomy and adenoidectomy	
Dental work	
Appendectomy or other surgical procedure	
Menstrual history (duration and amount)	
Medications (over-the-counter; prescription;	
aspirin, nonsteroidal anti-inflammatory drugs)	

Adapted from Hastings CA, Lubin BH. Blood. In: Rudolph AM, Kamei RK (eds), Rudolph's Fundamentals of Pediatrics, 2nd ed. Norwalk, CT: Appleton & Lange, 1998, pp 441–490.

PHYSICAL EXAMINATION

In addition to the routine examination, the skin should be scrutinized carefully for petechiae, purpura, and venous telangiectasias. The joints should be examined for swelling or chronic changes such as contractures or distorted appearance with asymmetry related to repeated bleeding episodes. Mucosal surfaces, such as the gingiva and nares, should be examined for bleeding.

LABORATORY EVALUATION

An attempt should be made to classify the bleeding abnormality as being related to primary or secondary hemostasis. The following screening tests provide information needed in the initial work-up of the child with a suspected bleeding diathesis.

COMPLETE BLOOD COUNT (WITH PLATELET COUNT AND PERIPHERAL BLOOD SMEAR ASSESSMENT)
Hemoglobin

- May be low due to excessive bleeding/blood loss.
- A primary bone marrow process, especially if more than one cell line is decreased, should be considered.

Platelets

Assess the number and morphology (size) of the platelets. For the thrombo-cytopenic patient, assessment of the platelet size can correlate with the underlying mechanism involved; that is, large platelets can be seen in an "active marrow" as associated with platelet consumption, destruction, or se-questration (immune thrombocytopenic purpura). Certain inherited dis-eases have large platelets, normal-sized platelets are seen in primary bone marrow suppression, and small-sized platelets can be seen in certain condi-tions such as the Wiskott-Aldrich syndrome.

PROTHROMBIN TIME/INTERNATIONAL NORMALIZED RATIO

Measurement of the prothrombin time (PT) evaluates the extrinsic system of coagulation. Factor VII is unique to the extrinsic pathway. Thus, in iso-lated factor VII deficiency, the PT is prolonged with a normal activated par-tial thromboplastin time (aPTT). Factor VII has a very short half-life, so the PT is one of the most sensitive measurements of oral anticoagulant therapy.

Variation in PT results can be minimized by reporting the PT as an Inter-national Normalized Ratio (INR). The INR is calculated as the patient PT/ control PT to the power of the International Sensitivity Index (ISI). The ISI corrects for the large variation in sensitivity of thromboplastin reagents to low plasma concentrations of some coagulation proteins. A normal value is 1.00 to 1.10. The INR is designed to be used with oral anticoagulant therapy.

ACTIVATED PARTIAL THROMBOPLASTIN TIME

The aPTT assesses the integrity of the intrinsic system of coagulation. De-pending on the laboratory methods, the aPTT will be normal with at least 30% activity of coagulation factors present. Some important considerations when interpreting an abnormal aPTT are listed below.

Sample Collection

Clots. Any small clots in the sample will give abnormal results.

Plasma Volume. The amount of anticoagulant must be corrected for the plasma volume. Thus, if the citrate tube is not completely filled, or the patient is extremely anemic or polycythemic (i.e., cyanotic congenital heart disease, chronic obstructive pulmonary disease, or cystic fibrosis), the sample will not be properly anticoagulated prior to testing.

Heparin Contamination

Heparin contamination is one of the most common causes of a prolonged aPTT. If the initial blood sample was obtained through a heparinized line, a peripheral sample may be indicated. The aPTT is widely used for monitor-ing heparin therapy, with a usual goal of obtaining a range of 1.5 to 2.5 times normal.

Age-Dependent Normal Values

A mildly prolonged aPTT is normal in the newborn infant because of immaturity of the coagulation system (reference tables are available for specific values). Most procoagulant and anticoagulant protein levels reach adult normal values by 6 months of age.

Inhibitor Versus Factor Deficiency

After exclusion of any of the above factors, a 1:1 mixing study should be performed to differentiate between an inhibitor and a factor deficiency as the cause of a prolonged aPTT. A 1:1 mixture of the patient's plasma and normal pooled plasma is prepared, and the aPTT is repeated. If the aPTT is not corrected, the presence of an inhibitor can be assumed. If the aPTT corrects, a deficiency of one or more coagulation factors probably exists, and specific factor assays should be performed.

Some inhibitors are time dependent, such as those to factor VIII, and an incubation period before the aPTT can assist in the diagnosis. The most frequent inhibitor encountered is heparin, and the second most frequent is the lupus anticoagulant. This inhibitor is present in 10% of patients with systemic lupus erythematosus, but the lupus anticoagulant is common in patients with no evidence of underlying collagen–vascular disease. Paradoxically, this anticoagulant is associated with clinical thrombosis rather than hemorrhage in up to 30% of patients. Therefore, an attempt to identify the nature of the anticoagulant is important. The anti-cardiolipin antibody test and lupus anticoagulant (anti-phospholipid antibody) test can help with this distinction.

THROMBIN TIME AND FIBRINOGEN

The thrombin time is abnormal when the plasma level of fibrinogen is decreased (hypofibrinogenemia or afibrinogenemia), when the fibrinogen is dysfunctional (dysfibrinogenemia), or when there are circulating anticoagulants (heparin) or fibrin degradation products. *A modified thrombin test, because of its extreme sensitivity to heparin, is frequently used as a control for heparin contamination in assessing the coagulation status of the patient.*

INTERPRETATION OF RESULTS

Abnormalities in one or more of the above screening tests will be noted with most bleeding disorders (Table 8–2). Further evaluation will often be necessary to specifically determine a diagnosis pending these results (Fig. 8–1). Of note, however, all the above tests are normal in patients with qualitative platelet disorders. As discussed in Chapter 9, von Willebrand disease can be characterized by fluctuating levels of the von Willebrand factor, and thus a normal screening aPTT is seen at times.

TABLE 8-2

INTERPRETATION OF LABORATORY STUDIES

PLATELET COUNT	PROTHROMBIN TIME (PT)	ACTIVATED PARTIAL THROMBOPLASTIN TIME (APTT)	DIFFERENTIAL DIAGNOSIS
Normal	Prolonged	Normal	Moderate liver disease Warfarin ingestion Factor VII deficiency, acquired or inherited
Normal	Normal	Prolonged	von Willebrand disease Heparin effect Factor VIII, IX, XI, or XII deficiency
Decreased	Prolonged	Prolonged	DIC Giant hemangioma CHD

Decreased	Normal	Normal	Lack of platelet production
			  Acute leukemia or other malignancy with marrow infiltration
			  Aplastic anemia
			  Thrombocytopenia
			    or
			Platelet consumption
			  ITP
			  Cyanotic CHD
			  NATP
			  Kasabach-Merritt syndrome

Normal	Prolonged	Prolonged	Severe liver disease (hepatitis, cirrhosis) Vitamin K deficiency Factor II, V, IX, or X deficiency High-dose heparin or warfarin Dysfibrinogenemia
Normal	Normal	Normal	von Willebrand disease Platelet dysfunction, qualitative Factor XIII deficiency Henoch-Schönlein purpura Connective tissue disease

Abbreviations: DIC = disseminated intravascular coagulation; CHD = congenital heart disease; ITP = immune thrombocytopenic purpura; NATP = neonatal alloimmune thrombocytopenia.

8

LABORATORY EVALUATION

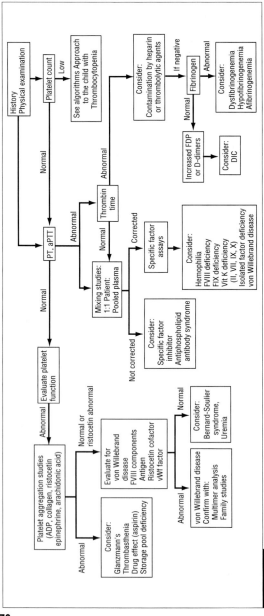

FIGURE 8-1

Laboratory evaluation of the child with a bleeding disorder. (Abbreviations: PT = prothrombin time; aPTT = activated partial thromboplastin time; ADP = adenosine diphosphate; F = factor; vWF = von Willebrand factor; FDP = fibrin degradation products; DIC = disseminated intravascular coagulation.) *(Adapted from Hastings CA, Lubin BH. Blood. In: Rudolph AM, Kamel RK [eds], Rudolph's Fundamentals of Pediatrics, 2nd ed. Norwalk, CT: Appleton & Lange, 1998, pp 441–490.)*

SUGGESTED READING

Hastings CA, Lubin BH. Blood. In: Rudolph AM, Kamei RK (eds), Rudolph's Fundamentals of Pediatrics, 2nd ed. Norwalk, CT: Appleton & Lange, 1998, pp 441–490.

Lanzkowsky P. Manual of Pediatric Hematology and Oncology, 3rd ed. San Diego: Academic Press, 2000.

Lusher JM. Approach to the bleeding patient. In: Nathan DG, Orkin SH (eds), Nathan and Oski's Hematology of Infancy and Childhood, 5th ed. Philadelphia: WB Saunders, 1998, pp 1574–1584.

von WILLEBRAND DISEASE

von Willebrand disease (vWD) is the most common inherited bleeding disorder, affecting 1 in every 200 to 500 individuals. vWD is usually inherited in an autosomal dominant manner, but at least two variants of this disorder have been recognized: a rare autosomal recessive form and an X-linked recessive type. vWD is a disorder or the protein vWf (von Willebrand factor), which is responsible for the adherence of platelets to damaged endothelium. Deficiency of this protein results in mucocutaneous bleeding and post-traumatic or postsurgical bleeding. vWD should be suspected in the patient with platelet-type bleeding and a family history of a bleeding diathesis.

vWf is a large, multimeric glycoprotein that is synthesized in megakaryocytes and endothelial cells. Desmopressin can induce the release of vWf from storage sites in the plasma and result in elevated circulating levels of vWf. This vWf binds platelet glycoprotein Ib, causing platelet activation and adherence to damaged endothelium. vWf also serves as a carrier protein for the plasma factor VIII molecule, and its absence results in a secondary deficiency of plasma factor VIII. Thus patients with severe vWD (type III) have a prolonged bleeding time and a prolonged activated partial thromboplastin time (aPTT) caused by a decrease in both vWf and factor VIII.

CLINICAL PRESENTATION

The clinical picture is variable, depending on whether the defect is a quantitative or qualitative deficiency of vWf. Males and females are similarly affected, and symptoms can be mild or as severe as hemophilia. There are several subtypes, categorized on the basis of factor VIII levels (antigen, ristocetin cofactor, vWf) and multimer structure.

In most cases of vWD, the bleeding is mild. Mucosal bleeding, such as epistaxis, gingival bleeding with toothbrushing, ecchymoses, or menorrhagia, is the classical symptom. The initial presentation, however, may be postoperative bleeding, such as following a tonsillectomy and adenoidectomy or dental extraction. In retrospect, the child who was thought to have normal childhood complaints (bruising and epistaxis) is realized to actually have a bleeding disorder. Recurrent or severe epistaxis, particularly in the older child or adult, is unusual and warrants investigation. It is important to obtain a thorough medical history of bleeding from the family (see Chapter 8) because this may provide clues. Often, the child is diagnosed with vWD and then a parent or siblings are found to have the disorder after screening.

In patients with mild vWD, the stress associated with serious operations or childbirth may preclude symptoms. vWf acts as an acute-phase reactant and can be elevated in certain states, such as postoperatively, in pregnancy, in liver disease, or in collagen–vascular disease. It can be reduced in hypothyroidism. Even the stress of phlebotomy is thought to increase the level of vWf, making it difficult to confirm the diagnosis even with repeat testing.

Neonates have elevated vWf levels following vaginal delivery, again making vWD difficult to diagnose in the neonatal period.

DIAGNOSIS

vWD can be difficult to diagnose because factor VIII levels, particularly in mild to moderate disease, can fluctuate with stress and result in either abnormal or normal screening tests by aPTT or bleeding time. Thus a normal aPTT or bleeding time does not rule out a diagnosis of vWD. Specific testing as described below must be performed for diagnosis, often on repeated occasions because of fluctuating levels. In the majority of cases, vWD can be diagnosed by evaluation of the results of the following four tests:

1. **Ristocetin cofactor** (functional activity of vWf): Ristocetin induces the binding of vWf to the glycoprotein Ib receptor on fixed platelets, thus the slope of the platelet agglutination curve correlates with the amount of plasma vWf.
2. **von Willebrand factor antigen** (vWf:Ag): Immunologic quantitation of vWf by either the quantitative immunoelectrophoretic assay (Laurell assay) or the enzyme-linked immunosorbent assay.
3. **Factor VIII coagulant** (F VIII:C): functional measurement of factor VIII that is carried in the circulation by vWf.
4. **Multimeric analysis:** an agarose gel electrophoretic study used to identify quantitative or qualitative multimer abnormalities. The most common type of vWD (type I) has a normal multimeric analysis.

TREATMENT

Treatment of vWD requires knowledge of the clinical subtype. Desmopressin is the treatment of choice in mild type I disease (65% to 80% of all cases) and may be of benefit with some of the other variants. Desmopressin is a safe and easy therapy to administer. It stimulates endogenous release of vWf, with most patients experiencing a 2- to 4-fold increase in their plasma vWf and factor VIII levels within 15 to 30 minutes of the infusion. The approximate half-life of these released factors is 12 hours. Occasionally, patients do not respond to this therapy (especially children younger than 18 months of age). The peak effect is observed in 30 to 60 minutes. A therapeutic trial of desmopressin is usually given to determine individual responsiveness to this therapy, with measurement of aPTT and factor VIII levels before and after administration.

A standard dose of 0.3 μg/kg is administered intravenously in 50 ml of normal saline over 15 to 30 minutes (10 ml in a child <10 kg). Alternatively, an intranasal form of desmopressin (Stimate, 1.5 mg/ml) may be used as a challenge or to treat bleeding in vWD. Though effective, there is some variability in response as a result of inconsistent absorption. The effective dose in adolescents and adults is 150 μg per nostril (total dose of 300 μg [two puffs]). Children weighing less than 50 kg should receive a total dose of 150 µg (one puff), though they should be old enough to cooperate with this therapy. The peak effect is observed 60 to 90 minutes after administration therapy. Care should be taken not to administer a dilute form of desmopressin nasal spray (0.1 mg/ml) developed for use in patients with diabetes insipidus.

Patients undergoing surgical procedures, including dental extractions, may need extended therapy to maintain increased levels of vWf and factor VIII levels until healing has occurred. Repeated infusions of desmopressin at 12- to 24-hour intervals are effective, but can result in tachyphylaxis. Pre- and postinfusion measurements of vWf or ristocetin cofactor should be done to establish continued clinical responsiveness. In patients whose levels of vWf have dropped to 15 to 20 U/dL and in the perioperative period, treatment with plasma-derived vWf/factor VIII may be needed.

With any vWD patient with severe bleeding manifestations or with desmopressin-unresponsive type II or type III disease, treatment with plasma-derived products is required. No vWf-containing concentrates are approved for the specific treatment of vWD. Most hemophilia treatment centers use these concentrates in an "off-label" manner. Clinical trials have demonstrated their efficacy in the cessation of bleeding related to vWD, but they are not approved by the Food and Drug Administration (FDA) for this disorder. Several products, including the human antihemophilic factor drugs Humate-P and Alphanate, are undergoing clinical trials for FDA approval. Treatment with factor concentrate is based on attaining a factor VIII level of 30% to 50%, with 1 IU/kg body weight of vWf required to increase the plasma level by 2 IU/dL. Cryoprecipitate contains adequate vWf levels but is not routinely used because it cannot be specifically treated to remove viruses. Its use should be reserved for emergencies. Plasma levels of either vWf or factor VIII should be about 100 U/dL preoperatively, and then be maintained above 50 U/dL for 3 to 7 days after major surgery.

Epistaxis is a common problem in vWD and can usually be controlled with local pressure (see Chapter 11). If uncontrolled, a single dose of desmopressin is usually effective to stop bleeding. Oral contraceptives have been very helpful in controlling menorrhagia. Minor surgical procedures, such as laceration repairs or dental extractions, can frequently be treated with a single infusion of desmopressin or factor concentrate along with **antifibrinolytic therapy** for 7 to 10 days. Two antifibrinolytic agents, aminocaproic acid and tranexamic acid, are available. The oral dose of aminocaproic acid is 100 to 200 mg/kg (maximum dose 10 g) initial dose, followed by 50 to 100 mg/kg/dose (maximum dose 5 g) every 6 hours. The dose of tranexamic acid is 25 mg/kg/dose every 6 to 8 hours. Both drugs are available in oral and intravenous forms. These drugs have been most successfully used to prevent hemorrhage for dental extractions. Tranexamic acid has also been shown to be effective when used topically, as in mouthwash.

In **type III** vWD, plasma vWf and factor VIII levels are excessively low (typically less than 5 U/dL) and desmopressin is usually ineffective. A therapeutic trial of desmopressin may be given because occasional patients may respond appropriately. These individuals are severely affected and may have spontaneous bleeding, including profound epistaxis or joint bleeding, such as seen in hemophilia. Such patients should be managed for bleeding similarly to patients with hemophilia, using factor VIII concentrates that contain high levels of vWf.

Patients with **type IIA** vWD have abnormally small vWf multimers, and desmopressin, though frequently effective, may have a transient effect at best. Serious bleeding should be treated with plasma-derived factor VIII/vWf concentrates. These patients may do well with desmopressin for the treatment of minor bleeds or dental extractions.

Type IIB vWD is often associated with mild thrombocytopenia resulting from platelet binding to an abnormal vWf molecule and rapid clearance. Stress can exacerbate the thrombocytopenia. Desmopressin is usually not given because of the potential for increased platelet activation and failure to demonstrate a therapeutic response. However, in mild bleeding desmopressin may be effective. For internal bleeding or surgery, patients should receive factor VIII/vWf concentrate. If profound thrombocytopenia exists, concomitant administration of platelets may be necessary.

As a general precaution, all children with bleeding disorders should be immunized with the hepatitis B vaccine, with boosters given at appropriate time intervals. These children have lifelong potential for receiving blood products. Also, it is generally recommended that children wear Medic Alert bracelets or have information readily available (at school, home, doctor's office) specifying the diagnosis and treatment for bleeding.

ACQUIRED VON WILLEBRAND DISEASE

vWD may be acquired in children who were previously normal. This is frequently a result of antibodies to vWf that neutralize its activity. Patients present with classical signs and symptoms of vWD, and their levels of vWf, vWf:Ag, and factor VIII are all markedly reduced. Inhibitors may occur in otherwise healthy individuals, but frequently are associated with an underlying immunologic disorder. Acquired vWD has been reported following viral infections and in association with Wilms' tumor. It may also occur in association with cardiac disease as a result of increased utilization of vWf. Desmopressin may induce a transient rise in vWf. Intravenous immune globulin may be beneficial in some cases. For serious bleeding, treatment with factor concentrate (high vWf content) should be given. The antibodies may disappear with control or resolution of the underlying disease.

SUGGESTED READING

Lanzkowsky P. Manual of Pediatric Hematology and Oncology, 3rd ed. San Diego: Academic Press, 2000.

Montgomery RR, Gill JC, Scott JP. Hemophilia and von Willebrand disease. In: Nathan DG, Orkin SH (eds), Nathan and Oski's Hematology of Infancy and Childhood, 5th ed. Philadelphia: WB Saunders, 1998, pp 1631–1659.

HEMOPHILIAS

HEMOPHILIA A AND B

Classical hemophilia, or **hemophilia A**, is the most common hereditary clotting factor deficiency, with an estimated incidence of 1 in 4000 males. The recessive gene is located on the X chromosome and linked closely to the genes for color blindness and glucose-6-phosphate dehydrogenase. The disorder results from the deficiency of the factor VIII antigen (factor VIII:Ag), a small subunit of the factor VIII molecule. Female carriers are usually unaffected, and the disease is seen almost exclusively in the male population.

Hemophilia B, or factor IX deficiency, is inherited as an X-linked recessive trait and is much less common than factor VIII deficiency, accounting for 12% of all hemophiliac patients. The clinical findings and initial evaluation are similar to factor VIII deficiency, although factor IX deficiency can be milder.

Clinically, the first indication that a bleeding disorder is present may be from hemorrhage after circumcision or separation of the umbilical cord. However, up to 70% of affected male infants have no difficulty during the neonatal period, and a negative history of bleeding after circumcision does not rule out the diagnosis of hemophilia. Mild hemophilia may go unsuspected for years until the patient experiences trauma or has a surgical procedure. Hemorrhage can occur spontaneously and be internal or external. Large hematomas can result in secondary conditions such as hemarthrosis, disability, and joint degeneration. Significant blood loss can occur with muscular bleeds, and the leading cause of death is intracranial hemorrhage.

DIAGNOSIS

The diagnosis of factor VIII deficiency should be suspected in males with bleeding characteristic of factor deficiency, a family history of males with bleeding diatheses, or abnormal clotting studies (prolonged activated partial thromboplastin time [aPTT]). It can be confirmed by specific factor assays. The frequency and severity of bleeding manifestations in a hemophiliac patient can be roughly predicted by the baseline factor level.

The factor (procoagulant) level is measured in comparison to a reference standard that is assumed to have a factor level of 100% (1.0 U/ml). In the normal individual, factor VIII and IX levels range from 50% to 200% (0.50 to 2.0 U/ml).

Disease severity is defined as **severe** (<2%), **moderate** (2% to 5%), and **mild** (>5%). Hemophilia A and B are clinically indistinguishable because both factors VIII and IX are essential factors in the intrinsic clotting pathway for activating factor X.

An infant with a suspected or known history of hemophilia should be carefully evaluated for an intracranial hemorrhage, particularly after a vaginal delivery. Initial studies can be performed in the newborn period on cord blood by screening with aPTT, recognizing that newborn normal values are slightly more elevated than in the adult (reference tables are available).

10

Although factor VIII levels in the newborn parallel adult values, factor IX levels are often lower initially until there is maturation of liver-produced proteins. Thus diagnosis of hemophilia B may be more difficult initially. Confirmatory studies should be performed on a sample obtained by venipuncture, if a cord blood sample was initially obtained. Use of arterial and femoral or jugular venous sites to obtain plasma samples should be avoided if possible.

TREATMENT

Treatment of patients with hemophilia and bleeding is by replacement of factor in a concentrated form. Many preparations are available, including recombinant products. Duration, frequency, and dosages of the treatments depend on the severity of the hemophilia and bleeding episode (see Chapter 11).

In all children with hemophilia, in addition to replacement of appropriate factor levels when bleeding has occurred and use of physical therapy programs to prevent or minimize chronic joint disease, comprehensive medical care must be given. Immunizations to prevent hepatitis B should be given as soon as possible after birth; appropriate consideration and screening procedures for human immunodeficiency virus, prophylactic dental care, and aggressive management of hemarthrosis are required. Emotional support is essential to assist patients and families to cope with the emotional and social burden imposed by the disease. Prevention of chronic joint complications is critical for the health and well-being of patients with hemophilia, and home care treatment should be used when possible.

Unfortunately, approximately 10% of patients with severe hemophilia develop antibody to administered concentrates containing the specific factor required for treatment. This prevents response to therapy and requires specific steps, such as consideration of immune suppressive therapy, exchange transfusion, administration of prothrombin complex, and, in most cases, administration of sufficient factor product to block circulating antibody and still provide procoagulant activity.

HEMOPHILIA C (FACTOR XI DEFICIENCY)

This coagulation defect is transmitted as an autosomal recessive trait and occurs in both sexes, primarily in patients of Jewish ancestry. The homozygotes can have severe factor XI deficiency, although the clinical manifestations are milder than those in patients with factor VIII or IX deficiency. Bleeding episodes can be managed by infusion of 10 ml/kg of fresh frozen plasma.

FACTOR XIII DEFICIENCY (FIBRIN-STABILIZING FACTOR)

This coagulation abnormality is unique in that the patient presents with bleeding soon after birth, similar to the types seen with classical hemophilia, but standard laboratory assays such as prothrombin time, aPTT, and thrombin time are normal. A high index of suspicion is essential to establish the diagnosis, which can be accomplished by determining the solubility of the patient's clot in 5 M urea. Normal clots are insoluble because of the action of fibrin-stabilizing factor. Clots from patients with this deficiency are readily dissolved. The disorder can be treated with plasma infusions.

OTHER RARE COAGULATION ABNORMALITIES

α_2-Antiplasmin deficiency, factor XII deficiency, prekallikrein (Fletcher's factor) deficiency, high-molecular-weight kininogen (Fitzgerald's factor) deficiency, hereditary afibrinogenemia or dysfibrinogenemia, and deficiencies of isolated prothrombin as well as factors V, VII, and X have all been identified using appropriate clotting measurements. Prekallikrein deficiency, high-molecular-weight kininogen deficiency, and factor XII deficiency all cause laboratory abnormalities but are not associated with clinical hemorrhage.

SUGGESTED READING

Montgomery RR, Cox JC, Scott JP. Hemophilia and von Willebrand disease. In: Nathan DG, Orkin SH (eds), Nathan and Oski's Hematology of Infancy and Childhood, 5th ed. Philadelphia: WB Saunders, 1998, pp 1631–1659.

10

OTHER RARE COAGULATION ABNORMALITIES

MANAGEMENT OF ACUTE HEMORRHAGE IN BLEEDING DIATHESES

COMPLICATIONS OF BLEEDING DIATHESES

11

HEMARTHROSES

Acute hemarthroses can begin in children as they become mobile. The knees and elbows initially with crawling, and then other joints (ankles, shoulders, hips, and wrists, in descending order), are targeted with increased mobility. The hands and spine are rarely involved. The initial signs of a hemarthrosis are vague and difficult to detect, especially early on in the nonverbal infant. Early, aggressive treatment of an acute hemarthrosis is recommended to relieve symptoms and, hopefully, prevent rebleed in the same joint, setting up the situation of a "target" joint. Treatment to achieve a factor level of 35% to 40% is recommended for an acute hemarthrosis. Retreatment for 2 to 5 days may be necessary to prevent the development of a target joint. Other important interventions for a hemarthrosis include initial immobilization and application of ice to the area or use of a Cryocuff. For particularly critical joints such as the shoulder or hip, where long-term consequences of avascular necrosis can be debilitating, a longer treatment course is recommended.

MUSCLE BLEEDS

Similar to hemarthroses, a muscle bleed should be promptly treated considering the immediate symptoms of pain and limitation of full mobility, as well as the potential long-term complications of permanent muscle contractures. An intramuscular bleed can be difficult to evaluate depending on the location of the muscle involved. It is important to exclude any potential neurovascular compromise. For most muscle bleeds, therapy to achieve a factor level of 30% to 40% is recommended.

Iliopsoas Bleed

An iliopsoas hemorrhage can be particularly devastating considering not only the long-term consequences, but additionally the potential large volume of blood loss that can occur acutely into this large muscle bed and into the retroperitoneal space. The presenting signs of groin or lower abdominal/upper thigh pain can be difficult to differentiate from a hip bleed. With an iliopsoas bleed, examination reveals inability to extend the hip, with normal internal and external hip rotation. Radiologic confirmation by ultrasound or computed tomography (CT) scan is often necessary for clinical correlation. Aggressive long-term therapy is required until there is evidence of clinical and radiologic improvement.

SOFT TISSUE HEMORRHAGE

Soft tissue hemorrhages do not require therapy unless their location is in close proximity to vital structures. For instance, a retropharyngeal bleed with potential airway compromise should be aggressively treated. Vigorous examination of the oropharynx with a tongue blade or other manipulations should be avoided to prevent this as an iatrogenic complication.

A **"straddle"** injury resulting in a hematoma of the perineal/perirectal area should be closely evaluated for neurologic compromise as evidenced by either bladder or bowel dysfunction.

HEMATURIA

Approximately two thirds of hemophiliacs will have at least one episode of hematuria. Usually these episodes are painless; thus, if there is severe pain associated with hematuria, a renal pelvic hematoma should be excluded.

Increased fluid intake and bed rest is recommended. Factor replacement may be warranted with persistent symptoms. Treatment with antifibrinolytic drugs is contraindicated given the risk of urinary obstruction.

NEUROLOGIC BLEEDING

An intracranial hemorrhage is the most serious complication in hemophilia. Central nervous system hemorrhages may occur without known antecedent trauma, and early symptoms may be minimal. The morbidity of those patients who survive is also high, with reports of mental retardation, seizure disorders, or motor impairment. Any history of head trauma should be considered emergent. A nonfocal neurologic examination does not exclude a diagnosis of an intracranial bleed because late bleeding after head trauma can occur, as long as 3 to 4 weeks after the initial trauma. A low index of suspicion should prompt a head CT and close neurologic observation. Immediate treatment to a factor level of 80% to 100% should be instituted until an intracranial bleed can be fully excluded. An intraspinal hemorrhage should be excluded with any back trauma or symptoms of a peripheral neuropathy. A lumbar puncture should *never* be performed in a hemophiliac without factor therapy to avoid this potential complication.

MUCOSAL MEMBRANE BLEEDING

Epistaxis is seen in hemophiliacs, more commonly in those with severe disease. Gastrointestinal bleeding can be seen as well but is atypical, and an underlying gastrointestinal lesion should be fully excluded. Intramural bleeding into the bowel wall can occur, with signs of severe pain and possible intestinal obstruction. Appropriate therapy may avoid an unnecessary laparotomy.

DENTAL BLEEDING

Prolonged gingival oozing is common after shedding of deciduous teeth, eruption of new teeth, or instrumentation. Treatment with antifibrinolytic medication is recommended for prolonged symptoms. Routine dental care is particularly important in the patient with a bleeding disorder, to prevent the need for restorative care in the future, for which extensive factor replacement therapy is often indicated. Regional block anesthesia should *never* be performed, especially without factor coverage, given the risk of nerve damage and bleeding into the floor of the mouth, with extension leading to airway compromise.

SURGICAL BLEEDING

A treatment plan for surgical procedures in the patient with coagulopathy should be carefully planned after evaluating the exact procedure to be performed, inhibitor status, response to therapy, and expected postoperative course.

TREATMENT

Usually, treatment becomes necessary when bleeding complications arise as the child becomes more mobile with increasing age. Some hemophilia treatment centers are investigating the use of **primary prophylaxis**, which involves regularly scheduled factor treatment prior to onset of recurrent bleeds and development of "target" joints. **Secondary prophylaxis**, which involves regular periodic factor treatment after an initial bleed to prevent development of a target joint, is advocated in specific individuals.

Treatment recommendations (Table 11–1) for the hemophiliac patient depend on several factors:

1. Type and severity of disease: mild, moderate, or severe factor VIII or IX deficiency
2. Location of bleed: site of bleed, proximity in and around vital structures, and consideration of long-term debilitating consequences
3. Therapy response: consideration of factor recovery/survival and inhibitor status

Instituting appropriate therapy as expeditiously as possible is important to prevent devastating immediate and long-term consequences for the hemophiliac patient. When prolonged periods of factor replacement are required, continuous infusion therapy is an alternative to bolus therapy, and is more physiologic and cost effective.

DESMOPRESSIN

Desmopressin (DDAVP) is a synthetic analogue of vasopressin that leads to endothelial release of factor VIII and von Willebrand factor, and can be a form of treatment and prophylaxis for the mild bleeding episodes in the patient with mild hemophilia A or von Willebrand disease. Because the individual response to this therapy is varied, a diagnostic trial with determination of pre– and post–factor VIII or ristocetin factor response is strongly

TABLE 11-1

TREATMENT OF SPECIFIC HEMORRHAGES IN HEMOPHILIA

TYPE OF BLEED	LOCATION	DOSAGE (F VIII)	DOSAGE (F IX)
Mild	Epistaxis	*Local pressure 15–20 minutes. Pack as needed. Antifibrinolytic therapy.*	
		20 U/kg if above fails	30 U/kg if above fails (4 hours after an antibrinolytic dose)
Moderate	Hemarthrosis	20 U/kg	30 U/kg
	Intramuscular		
		Remove loose tooth.	
	Mouth, deciduous tooth, tooth extraction	20 U/kg	30 U/kg; antifibrinolytic 4–6 hours after concentrate
		Bed rest, increased fluid intake (1–1½ × maintenance). If not controlled in 1–2 days:	
	Hematuria	20 U/kg	30 U/kg
		If not controlled:	
		Prednisone (2 mg/kg/day × 2 days)	Prednisone (1 mg/kg/day × 3 days)
Severe	Illiopsoas	50 U/kg; then 25 U/kg q12h; treat 10–14 days	80 U/kg; then 20–40 U/kg q12–24h; treat 10–14 days
Life threatening	Central nervous systems	50 U/kg, then continuous infusion of 2–3 U/kg/hour to maintain F VIII >100 U/dL for 24 hours; titrate to keep levels >30–50 U/dL for 10–14 days	80 U/kg, then 20–40 U/kg q12–24h to maintain F IX >30–40 U/dL for 10–14 days
	Major surgery/trauma		
	Airway obstruction		
	Gastrointestinal		

recommended before its use. Even if a response to intravenous DDAVP has been noted, response to the intranasal form of DDAVP (Stimate) should be also documented because of variable absorption. An individual usually responds similarly to DDAVP on subsequent exposures; however, after repeated doses, tachyphylaxis can develop. Thus recommendations are that it not be used more than once daily, and, if used repeatedly, especially in the postoperative (dental) situation, levels be monitored for effect.

Dosage
- Parenteral: 0.3 μg/kg in 50 ml normal saline over 20 to 30 minutes for children greater than 10 kg (dilute in 10 ml for children less than 10 kg)
- Intranasal: 150 μg (1 puff) for children less than 50 kg; 300 μg (1 puff in each nostril) for children 50 kg or greater

Side Effects
The primary side effects of DDAVP are headaches and facial flushing. Hyponatremia has been observed in patients receiving repeated doses of DDAVP or large volumes of oral or intravenous fluids. Hyponatremic seizures have been reported in children under 2 years of age.

Precautions
Recommendations during the administration of DDAVP are as follows:

1. Place the patient on mild fluid restriction; avoid oral or intravenous fluids containing low concentrates of electrolytes
2. Monitor urinary output

FACTOR REPLACEMENT THERAPY
Many recombinant products are now available for treatment of factor VIII and IX deficiency. Factor vials come in preset amounts. Use vials that come closest to the calculated target dose. Use the whole vial, because factor is expensive and is not uniformly dispersed in suspension. Ideally, patients should have a supply of factor available at home, to be administered whenever necessary.

Dosage
- Units (of factor VIII) = weight (kg) × % rise of factor VIII level × 0.5
- For factor IX replacement, multiply above value × 2 (for Bene FIX, multiply × 2.4)

ANTIFIBRINOLYTIC THERAPY
Antifibrinolytic therapy can additionally be used for control of mucosal membrane bleeding, particularly in the oral mucosa, where the salivary enzymes possess fibrinolytic activity. Use of antifibrinolytic agents for bleeding of other mucosal surfaces, such as the nasal and gastrointestinal mucosa, has not been studied extensively, and use is contraindicated for bleeding in

the urinary tract. After factor VIII replacement or desmopressin, use of antifibrinolytic agents for 7 to 10 days postbleed has significantly decreased the need for subsequent treatment. Two antifibrinolytic agents used are aminocaproic acid 50 to 100 mg/kg/dose (maximum 5 g) PO q6h or tranexamic acid 25 mg/kg/dose PO q6–8h. Both of these agents are available in a parenteral form. Use of antifibrinolytic agents with activated prothrombin complex concentrate (APCC) should be avoided (see below).

INHIBITORS

Up to 25% of severe hemophilia A patients develop factor VIII inhibitors, which are neutralizing antibodies that inactivate the procoagulant activity of exogenously administered factor. The frequency of inhibitor development to factor IX is much lower. Identifying the presence of an inhibitory antibody to factor VIII or IX is crucial because this will influence therapeutic response. An inhibitor can be identified either clinically, when there is a poor response to replacement therapy, or during routine screening evaluation. Inhibitors most commonly develop in severe hemophiliacs, often after the first 9 to 11 exposures. The Bethesda Inhibitor Assay (BIA) is the most commonly used measurement of the inhibitor titer. One Bethesda unit is the dilution of plasma that inhibits 50% of normal factor VIII or IX after incubation for 2 hours. Thus, if a 1:10 dilution of the patient plasma inactivates 50% of the normal plasma factor level by 25% to 75%, the result is reported as 10 Bethesda units.

Patients with inhibitors can be divided into

1. Low-titer responders (BIA <10). These patients have a lower titer inhibitor for which treatment with factor concentrate at higher doses usually can be used by saturating out the antibody.
2. High-titer responders (BIA >10). These patients have a higher titer inhibitor with an anamnestic response with subsequent exposure to factor. These high-titer inhibitors are less commonly transient, and are difficult to eradicate. Often alternative forms of therapy besides factor VIII replacement are required, as discussed below.

TREATMENT IN PATIENTS WITH HIGH-TITER INHIBITORS
Activated Prothrombin Complex Concentrates

Two commercially available APCCs, Autoplex and FEIBA (Factor Eight Inhibitor Bypassing Activity), contain activated factors VII and X, as well as thrombin and factor IX, which theoretically work by bypassing factor VIII, leading to the creation of a fibrin clot.

The initial recommended dosage is 75 U/kg, which can be repeated in 6 to 12 hours. When repeated doses are used, monitoring for disseminated intravascular coagulation should be emphasized. Antifibrinolytic therapy should not be used concurrently with APCCs.

Porcine Factor VIII Concentrate

Porcine factor VIII is another alternative therapy for the patient with a high-titer inhibitor. Prior to using this product, measurement of an anti–porcine factor VIII antibody should be obtained to rule out an anamnestic response. The recommended starting dose is 100 to 150 U/kg/dose.

Recombinant Factor VIIa

A recombinant activated factor VII concentrate (NovoSeven) can be administered to achieve hemostasis in patients with high-titer inhibitors. The initial dose is 90 µg/kg every 2 hours until hemostasis is achieved. Subsequent infusions and duration of therapy are dependent on the clinical response and severity of bleeding.

Intravenous Gamma Globulin

Intravenous gamma globulin has been shown to reduce, and occasionally eradicate, factor VIII inhibitors in some patients. This has been particularly true in acquired autoantibody situations.

Immune Tolerance

Some hemophilia treatment centers are using immune tolerance protocols to eradicate or decrease inhibitor titers. Initially, high doses of factor VIII (100 U/kg q12h) are administered over prolonged periods of time. During this time, patients may need to be treated with other factor products for bleeds.

Other Therapies

Other therapies reported to treat inhibitors include plasmapheresis (in combination with factor VIII concentrates and/or intravenous gamma globulin) and immune suppression with short-term steroids, alone or in combination with cytotoxic agents (e.g., cyclophosphamide, cyclosporine, α-interferon, or vincristine).

EPISTAXIS

Epistaxis is an acute hemorrhage from the nostril, nasal cavity, or nasopharynx. Hemorrhage more often occurs anteriorly, in the nasal septum, from the Kiesselbach plexus near the nasal vestibule or anterior to the inferior turbinate. Posterior hemorrhage originates in the posterior nasal cavity or nasopharynx, usually below the posterior half of the inferior turbinate or roof of the nasal cavity.

Successful management of epistaxis is based on location of the bleeding, and identification and treatment of a possible underlying disorder.

ASSESSMENT OF EPISTAXIS

1. Is bleeding bilateral or unilateral? Unilateral bleeding suggests anterior epistaxis.
2. What is the duration of nosebleed?

3. Is bleeding spontaneous or associated with trauma?
4. Is there any underlying bleeding diathesis? Medications? Thrombocytopenia?

MANAGEMENT OF EPISTAXIS

1. Place the patient in a sitting position to decrease venous pressure or, if the patient is recumbent in bed, turn the head to the side. Keep the head higher than the level of the heart. Do not allow the patient to lie flat.
2. Flex the patient's neck anteriorly, with the chin touching the chest.
3. With the thumb and index finger, pinch the soft parts of the nose. Hold pressure firmly over the lower half of the nose. Avoid compressing the upper half of the nose.
4. Hold pressure for **20 minutes** with the head in a flexed position. If manual pressure is stopped momentarily to examine or change dressings, the 20-minute digital pressure will likely need to start again. Pressure and time allow for clot formation to occur.
   a. If bleeding continues, reassess location of digital pressure and reapply.
   b. If bleeding stops and recurs, repeat manual pressure for 20 minutes.
   c. If bleeding continues reapply digital pressure for 20 minutes.
5. Advise the patient not to blow the nose for at least 12 hours to avoid dislodging the clot.
6. Nasal packing may be indicated if the source of bleeding is not well visualized or bleeding is profuse. Types of packing include compressed sponge, Vaseline gauze packing, gelfoam, or topical thrombin packing.
   a. Compressed sponges are compressed when dry and expand when wetted. The expansion produces active and passive absorption and places gentle pressure on the mucosa. The nasal sponge should fit snugly through the naris and be placed along the floor of the nasal cavity. Sponges are easy to insert and can be removed with little discomfort. Neosporin can be applied to the sponge for ease of insertion and to act as an antimicrobial agent. Topical thrombin powder (a vasoconstrictor) applied to the inserted end of the sponge can provide additional hemostasis.
   b. Anterior packs may be left in place for 1 to 5 days, though they should be removed within 24 hours in an immune-compromised patient because of the risk of infection.
   c. Humidification and nasal saline spray can help avoid drying and crusting of the oral mucous membranes as a result of mouth bleeding.
   d. Broad-spectrum antibiotics, to cover skin flora as well, should be considered in patients who are immune suppressed with a nasal pack in place.

e. Vaseline gauze packing, when placed correctly and snugly, is a reliable means of packing.

f. Packing may be soaked in 4% topical cocaine or a solution of 4% lidocaine and topical epinephrine (1:1000) to provide local anesthesia and vasoconstriction.

7. Cauterization may be necessary, especially if the area of bleeding can be identified.

8. If the patient has a known underlying acquired or inherited bleeding diathesis, other therapies may include DDAVP and an antifibrinolytic for von Willebrand disease or hemophilia, or platelet transfusion for thrombocytopenia (lack of production) or platelet dysfunction.

9. Transfusion of red blood cells may be indicated in cases of excessive blood loss (see Chapter 5 for guidelines).

10. An ear, nose, and throat specialist may be needed to assist with cases of excess blood loss or continued or repeat epistaxis.

11. Laboratory studies to consider include complete blood count, platelet count, prothrombin time, activated partial thromboplastin time, and type and cross. If excessive blood loss is thought to have occurred, repeat the hemoglobin in 1 to 2 hours.

SUGGESTEDED READING

Lanzkowsy P. Manual of Pediatric Hematology and Oncology, 3rd ed. San Diego: Academic Press, 2000.

Montgomery RR, Gill JC, Scott JP. Hemophilia and von Willebrand disease. In: Nathan DG, Orkin SH (eds), Nathan and Oski's Hematology of Infancy and Childhood, 5th ed. Philadelphia: WB Saunders, 1998, pp 1631–1659.

THE CHILD WITH THROMBOSIS

EVALUATION AND MANAGEMENT OF THE CHILD WITH THROMBOPHILIA

Venous thromboembolism has only recently been recognized as a rapidly increasing secondary complication in children being treated for serious, life-threatening primary diseases. There is still limited information on the relative importance of congenital and acquired risk factors, appropriate diagnostic tests, and optimal use of antithrombotic agents for the prevention and treatment of venous thromboembolism. Most recommendations are extrapolated from adult trials; however, optimal prevention and treatment in pediatric patients may differ for several reasons. These include physiologic age-dependent differences in the hemostatic system that influence the risk for venous thromboembolism, differing underlying etiologies and location of clots, and differing responses to antithrombotic agents.

Patients with a tendency to thrombosis are defined as having thrombophilia. Thrombophilia is usually suspected in patients with one or more of the following clinical features: idiopathic thrombosis, thrombosis at a young age, family history, recurrent thrombosis, or thrombosis at an unusual site. The incidence of venous thromboembolism is estimated at 53/100,000 hospitalized children and 240/100,000 hospitalized neonates. The greatest risk for thrombosis is in infancy and the teen years, usually in association with acquired prothrombotic conditions.

ACQUIRED RISK FACTORS

The single most common acquired risk factor for venous thromboembolism is the presence of a central venous catheter. Other acquired risk factors include trauma, surgery, nephrotic syndrome, diabetes, inflammatory bowel disease, collagen–vascular disease, and malignancy (acute leukemia in association with the use of asparaginase).

Children may develop thrombosis in any vein. The most common sites are the large proximal veins of the upper and lower extremities. Unusual sites for thrombosis include the renal vein, portal vein, and pulmonary vessels. Many clots are related to the presence of central venous catheters, which are primarily located in the upper venous system. Symptoms of thrombosis include failure to aspirate blood or flush the line, swelling, pain, superior vena cava syndrome, chylothorax, recurrent bacteremia, and pulmonary embolus (PE). Chronic thrombosis can result in development of collateral circulation in the neck, chest, arm, and abdomen.

Several variables affect the incidence of central venous catheter–related deep venous thrombosis (DVT), such as the presence of an underlying disease, damage to the vessel wall with insertion, use of large catheters in small veins, duration of use, and injection of potentially thrombogenic substances (such as blood products and hyperalimentation). Many clots are asymptomatic. The frequency of thrombosis may be related to the sensitivity of the radiographic method for screening or evaluation.

PROTHROMBOTIC DISORDERS

There are several congenital and acquired prothrombotic disorders that are linked to thromboembolism during childhood (Table 12–1). The most well characterized are the deficiencies in the naturally occurring anticoagulants antithrombin III (AT III), protein C, and protein S. These deficiencies may be genetic or acquired, such as in consumptive processes (disseminated intravascular coagulation, clots, hemorrhage, inflammatory states, use of oral anticoagulants). Two recently recognized, and surprisingly common, genetic prothrombotic conditions are the factor V Leiden gene mutation and the prothrombin gene mutation. The factor V Leiden mutation is a result of a single point mutation causing the activated procoagulant factors V and VIII to become more resistant to inactivation by protein C. This results in protein C resistance. This mutation is now believed to be the most common inherited risk factor for development of venous thromboembolism. Another cause of activated protein C resistance is inheritance of the prothrombin gene mutation at 20210. It is recognized as the second most common inherited defect linked to venous thromboembolism in adults. This association in children has also been reported but requires further study. Other hereditary deficiencies causing thrombosis are hypofibrinogenemia, dysfibrinogenemia, homocystinuria (often seen with methylene tetrahydrofolate reductase deficiency), and heparin cofactor II deficiency.

Conditions in which coagulation factor deficiencies are present either because of lack of production or increased consumption include vitamin K deficiency (newborn, liver disease, sepsis, chronic illness, malnutrition, prolonged antibiotic use), congenital heart disease with associated polycythemia, and Kasabach-Merritt syndrome. Hypofibrinogenemia may be acquired secondary to consumptive states or decreased production, such as

---

TABLE 12–1

ALTERATIONS OF COAGULATION PROTEINS ASSOCIATED WITH A PROTHROMBOTIC STATE

Factor V Leiden mutation (activated protein C resistance)
Prothrombin gene 20210 gene mutation
Antithrombin III deficiency
Protein C deficiency
Protein S deficiency
Homocystinuria (methylene tetrahydrofolate reductase mutation)
Plasminogen deficiency
Dysfibrinogenemia/hypofibrinogenemia
Lupus anticoagulant

Adapted from Hastings CA, Lubin BH. Blood. In Rudolph AM, Kamei RK (eds), Rudolph's Fundamentals of Pediatrics, 3rd ed. Norwalk, CT: Appleton & Lange, 2002 (in press).

seen with the use of asparaginase in the treatment of acute lymphocytic leukemia.

HISTORY AND PHYSICAL EXAM

Evaluation of the child with thrombosis (Fig. 12–1) begins with a complete history. An assessment should consider the presence of prothrombotic stimuli such as trauma, surgery, immobilization, catheterization, and any underlying medical or inflammatory condition. The medication history should be reviewed, including an inquiry about the use of estrogens or oral contraceptives. An extensive family history should include an assessment of family members with venous thromboembolism or known congenital thrombophilia.

The physical examination should be complete, with a careful assessment of the skin and any catheter sites. Patients may have subtle signs or symptoms, even with such conditions as pulmonary emboli, renal vein thrombosis, and portal vein thrombosis. Clinically, there may be pain, swelling, warmth, or erythema in the area of the clot, especially if the clot is in an extremity. A clot in the upper venous system may lead to signs of superior vena cava syndrome.

The presence of a thrombus should be confirmed radiographically. Typically, in pediatric patients less invasive means of diagnosis are used. These diagnostic methods include Doppler ultrasound, computed tomography (CT), impedance plethysmography, venography, and magnetic resonance imaging.

GUIDELINES FOR ANTICOAGULATION THERAPY FOR VENOUS THROMBOEMBOLISM IN CHILDREN

The general principles for the treatment of thromboembolism incorporate heparin for treatment and prophylaxis. Additionally, acute events should be treated with a thrombolytic agent. Acute events are defined as likely occurring with hours to 3 to 5 days. When thrombolytic therapy is initiated early, there is a good chance the clot will be completely lysed. The most commonly used thrombolytic agents are tissue plasminogen activator t-PA (Alteplase) and urokinase. t-PA should be given at a rate of 0.1–0.5 mg/kg/hour IV for 6 hours (see Formulary for dosing guidelines). Plasminogen levels should be monitored, and replacement with fresh frozen plasma may be necessary. If urokinase is used, the standard dose is a loading dose of 4400 U/kg IV over 10 minutes followed by 4400 U/kg/hour for 6 hours. Heparin (20 U/kg/hour) should be given concomitantly with the thrombolytic agent.

Careful monitoring of the patient should be done and includes laboratory assessment with prothrombin time (PT), activated partial thromboplastin time (aPTT), fibrinogen, and fibrin degradation products or D-dimers prior to therapy and every 6 hours. Fibrinogen, AT III, and plasminogen levels in addition to the platelet count should be checked prior to therapy and at least

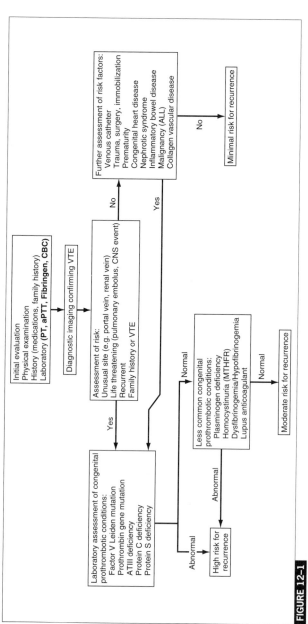

FIGURE 12-1

Evaluation of the child with venous thromboembolism. (Abbreviations: PT = prothrombin time; aPTT = activated partial thromboplastin time; CBC = complete blood count; VTE = venous thromboembolism; CNS = central nervous system; AT III = antithrombin III; MTHFR = methylene tetrahydrofolate reductase; ALL = acute lymphoblastic leukemia.) (Adapted from Hastings CA, Lubin BH. Blood. In: Rudolph AM, Kamei RK (eds). Rudolph's Fundamentals of Pediatrics, 3rd ed. Norwalk, CT: Appleton & Lange, 2002 [in press].)

daily during the infusions because replacement may be necessary. An objective diagnostic test (CT, ultrasound, or dye study) should be done following 6 hours of t-PA or urokinase infusion. If no response (clinical or radiographic) is noted, a repeat infusion of t-PA or urokinase should be considered. Minor bleeding may occur (i.e., oozing from venipuncture sites), but major bleeding would necessitate termination of thrombolytic and heparin therapies. If needed, the fibrinolytic process can be reversed with aminocaproic acid, 100 mg/kg (maximum 5 g) bolus, then 30 mg/kg/hour (maximum 1.25 g/hour) until the bleeding stops. Protamine sulfate may be required to reverse the heparin effect.

Standard heparin is part of a classical regimen for the treatment of acute venous thromboembolism. Heparin complexes to the physiologic inhibitor AT III and accelerates the inhibition of thrombin and other coagulant proteins. It is therefore important to ensure adequate levels of AT III when administering heparin. There are several problems with the use of standard heparin in children. These include its rapid clearance, low AT III levels in the first few months of life, greater variability in dosing compared to adults, and lack of clinical trials assessing the optimal target aPTT range for the prevention and treatment of venous thromboembolism.

Heparin is given as a loading dose of 75 mg/kg IV over 10 minutes, followed by a maintenance dose of 20 U/kg/hour in children over 1 year of age and 25 U/kg/hour in children under 1 year of age. It is given for a minimum of 5 days, and up to 10 to 14 days for extensive DVT or PE. Laboratory monitoring may be with anti–factor Xa levels (therapeutic range 0.30 to 0.70 U/ml) or with aPTT levels (to 150% of normal). Complications of heparin therapy include bleeding, heparin-induced thrombocytopenia (HIT), and osteoporosis. Oral anticoagulation (warfarin) should overlap for 4 to 5 days, with therapeutic International Normalized Ratios of 2 to 3 on 2 successive days.

Low-molecular-weight heparin (LMWH) is a recent therapeutic option rapidly gaining popularity because of its ease of use and fewer complications, especially in pediatrics. The starting dose is 1 mg/kg every 12 hours subcutaneously. Infants may require higher doses. Anti–factor Xa levels are monitored and should be drawn 4 hours after the injection, with a therapeutic range of 0.5 to 1.0 U/ml. LMWH can be used both in the acute therapeutic regimen and as prophylaxis.

The decision regarding who should receive prophylactic anticoagulation, when, and for how long should be made after considering risk factors, family history, age at presentation, site of the clot (life threatening?), and documentation of a congenital defect predisposing to thrombophilia. Patients at the highest risk for thrombosis are those with recurrent clots and the presence of an ongoing risk factor. These patients should receive anticoagulation indefinitely. Moderate risk factors are two or more idiopathic clots in children, young age, unusual site, familial, carriers of known thrombophilic conditions and a family history of clotting, or thromboembolism following a trivial provocation such as trauma, surgery, immobilization, or estrogen therapy. Prophylaxis in these patients should be limited to a defined risk period, usually 3 to 6 months, though, if the event was life threatening, there should be consideration for indefinite anticoagulation. The lowest risk patients are those with thromboembolism following no known provocation, with no family history and no known thrombophilic condition. These patients should receive short-term prophylaxis (less than 3 months) following treatment for a venous thromboembolism.

LOW-MOLECULAR-WEIGHT HEPARIN THERAPY

The following are guidelines for initiating and monitoring LMWH therapy. Modifications for individual clinical circumstances may be necessary.

Therapeutic Options

Two LMWHs have been studied in children, enoxaparin and reviparin. A pediatric hematology consultation is advised.

Indications

The use of LMWHs should be considered in neonates, any child requiring anticoagulation and deemed to be at risk for hemorrhage, and children in whom venous access for administration and monitoring of standard heparin therapy is difficult. Other situations may warrant the use of LMWH.

Dose

The dose of LMWH is dependent on age and use of LMWH as either treatment or prophylaxis. Beginning doses of enoxaparin are as follows:

	Age	
	<2 Months	*2 Months–18 Years*
Treatment dose	1.5 mg/kg/dose q12h	1.0 mg/kg/dose q12h
Prophylactic dose	0.75 mg/kg/dose q12h	0.5 mg/kg/dose q12h

The usual maximum dose is 2.0 mg/kg/dose BID. Doses should then be titrated by monitoring levels.

Monitoring

1. Prior to the initiation of LMWH therapy, obtain a complete blood count, PT, and aPTT.
2. In treating acute DVT or PE, encourage mobilization as tolerated.
3. Avoid aspirin or other antiplatelet drugs during heparin therapy. If analgesia is required, suggest acetaminophen.
4. Avoid IM injections and arterial punctures during anticoagulation.
5. Regularly measure platelet counts. If the platelet count drops below 100×10^9/L on day 5 or greater of initial LMWH therapy, or any day of LMWH therapy if the patient received heparin therapy in the last 3 months, consider testing for HIT. HIT is rarely due to LMWH.

6. Do blood work after the drug is administered and draw the sample from a fresh venipuncture. There must be **no heparin contamination** (e.g., from an arterial line).

7. On day 1 and/or day 2, draw a blood sample 4 to 6 hours after the SQ administration of LMWH. If therapeutic, a weekly check on the anti–factor Xa level is usually sufficient.

8. Aim for a therapeutic anti–factor Xa level for **treatment** of **0.5 to 1.0 U/mL**.

9. Aim for a therapeutic anti-factor Xa level for **prophylactic therapy** of **0.1 to 0.3 U/mL**.

10. For patients on long-term LMWH therapy (>3 months), consider bone densitometry studies at baseline and then at regular intervals (approximately every 6 months) to assess for possible osteoporosis.

11. If the patient has a lupus anticoagulant, remember that one cannot rely on the aPTT; monitor heparin (anti–factor Xa) levels.

Length of Therapy

The duration of LMWH therapy is dependent upon the primary problem. For DVT in children, LMWH is usually administered for a minimum of 7 days or for a full 3 to 6 months of therapy, instead of an oral anticoagulant. If an oral anticoagulant is used, it can usually be instituted on day 1 or 2 of heparin therapy.

- **Note:** If the thrombus is extensive or massive PE is present, administer LMWH for 7 to 14 days and begin warfarin therapy on day 5.
- **Note:** Newborns may be treated for 10 to 14 days with LMWH alone, and either receive no anticoagulants with close monitoring using objective tests, or carefully monitored warfarin therapy. This decision should be individualized following consultation with the pediatric hematologist. If the platelet count is less than 150×10^9/L or bleeding occurs, reassess.

Antidote

If anticoagulation with LMWH needs to be discontinued for clinical reasons, termination of the SQ injection will usually suffice. If an immediate effect is required, protamine sulfate has been shown to completely reverse LMWH.

The dose of protamine sulfate is dependent on the dose of LMWH used and the time of administration. If protamine is given within 3 to 4 hours of the LMWH, then a maximal neutralizing dose is **1 mg of protamine per 100 units (1 mg) of LMWH (most recent dose) over 10 minutes**. The protamine should be administered IV and over a 10-minute period, because rapid infusion can cause hypotension. Consultation with a pediatric hematologist is advised prior to this treatment.

12

ANTICOAGULATION THERAPY FOR VENOUS THROMBOEMBOLISM

Accumulation of LMWH

There is some evidence that LMWH may accumulate in the body over time, thereby changing dosing requirements. For patients on long-term therapy (>4 weeks), this possibility should be assessed. One approach is to measure an anti–factor Xa level 4 hours following the morning injection, every 2 weeks. If the level is greater than 1.0 U/mL, consult the hematologist. Discontinue LMWH 24 to 48 hours prior to a surgical procedure.

SUGGESTED READING

Andrew M, deVeber G. Pediatric Thromboembolism and Stroke Protocols. New York: BC Decker, 1997.

Andrew M, Montagle PT, Brooker L. Thromboembolic Complications During Infancy and Childhood. New York: BC Decker, 2000.

Hastings CA, Lubin BH. Blood. In: Rudolph AM, Kamei RK (eds), Rudolph's Fundamentals of Pediatrics, 2nd ed. Norwalk, CT: Appleton & Lange, 1998, pp 441–490.

Massicotte MP. Low-molecular-weight heparin therapy in children. J Pediatr Hematol Oncol 12:189–194, 2001.

NEUTROPENIA

Neutropenia is a condition in which inadequate numbers of granulocytes are present. Normal neutrophil counts vary by age and race. The absolute neutrophil count (ANC) is found by multiplying the white blood cell count (WBC) by the total percentage of bands plus segmented (mature) neutrophils:

$$ANC = WBC \times \% \text{ neutrophils (bands + segmented forms)}$$

Mild neutropenia is defined as an ANC of 1000 to 1500 cells/μl, moderate neutropenia is an ANC of 500 to 1000 cells/μl, and severe neutropenia is an ANC below 500 cells/μl. This division into three categories is useful for determining the individual's risk for infection and the urgency of medical intervention. In severely neutropenic patients, endogenous bacteria are the most frequent pathogens, but neutropenic hosts often become colonized with a variety of nosocomial organisms.

Susceptibility to bacterial infection in neutropenic patients is quite variable and depends on the cause of the neutropenia and other associated problems. Many patients with chronic neutropenia have an elevated circulating monocyte count, which provides limited protection against pyogenic organisms. Patients who are neutropenic as a result of cytotoxic therapy (e.g., chemotherapy, radiation) may be at an increased risk of infection because of the rate of decline of the neutrophil count, even before the ANC falls below 500 cells/μl. Additionally, these patients can have altered phagocytic function related to their therapy and defects in cell-mediated, humoral, and macrophage–monocyte immunity. Malnutrition, splenectomy, and increased exposure to pathogens further weaken the host. All these factors must be taken into consideration in assessing the patient with neutropenia.

Neutropenia may be caused by defects in myelopoiesis, congenital or acquired, or may be secondary to factors extrinsic to the bone marrow. Intrinsic defects of myelopoiesis are rare, but should still be included in the differential diagnosis of a newly identified patient with neutropenia, especially an infant.

CHRONIC BENIGN NEUTROPENIA OF CHILDHOOD

A particular group of children with chronic idiopathic neutropenia likely represents several poorly understood disorders. Many of these children have a benign course, hence the name *chronic benign neutropenia of childhood*. They often have mild to moderate neutropenia; the susceptibility to infection is roughly proportionate to the degree of neutropenia. The blood neutrophil count remains stable over years, and in a subset of children becomes elevated in response to an infection. Spontaneous remissions after 2 to 4 years have been reported. Some cases appear to be familial. Affected individuals have normal life expectancies. Evaluation of the bone marrow shows decreased myelopoiesis (often with monocytosis), and there is considerable variability in the stage at which maturation is arrested. These patients are at low risk for development of serious infections, and no treatment is required except during infectious episodes.

ANCs are significantly lower in African-Americans than in whites. The explanation for this difference is unclear. ANCs may be as low as 800/μl, yet they are not associated with infection, because an increase in ANC occurs in response to infection. Furthermore, the bone marrow aspirate is normal with respect to myelopoiesis. Red cell and platelet counts are also normal. If the history for infections is unremarkable, chronic neutropenia with counts over 500/μl in African-Americans requires no further investigation. If bacterial infections are present, these patients should have a complete evaluation of neutropenia.

EXTRINSIC CAUSES OF NEUTROPENIA

REPLACEMENT OF BONE MARROW
Replacement of the bone marrow (as occurs with hematologic malignancies, glycogen storage disease, granulomas associated with infection, and fibrosis related to chemical or radiation injury or osteoporosis) results in neutropenia. Frequently, the erythroid and megakaryocytic lines are also affected. Ineffective granulopoiesis can be seen in states of vitamin deficiency (vitamin B_{12} or folate), malnutrition (anorexia nervosa and marasmus), copper deficiency, and the Chédiak-Higashi syndrome.

VIRAL INFECTION
The most common cause of transient neutropenia in childhood is viral infection. Viruses known to cause neutropenia include hepatitis A and B, influenza A and B, measles, rubella, varicella, and respiratory syncytial virus. Neutropenia corresponds to the period of acute viremia–the first 24 to 48 hours of the illness, lasting up to 1 week. Neutropenia occurring 1 to 2 weeks after viremia suggests an immune-mediated mechanism of neutrophil destruction or sequestration, and the presence of antineutrophil antibodies can often be detected.

BACTERIAL SEPSIS
Bacterial sepsis is one of the more serious causes of neutropenia. Phagocytosis of microbes leads to release of toxic metabolites, which then activate the complement system, inducing neutrophil aggregation and adherence of leukocytes to the pulmonary capillary bed. Tumor necrosis factor and interleukin-1, released by macrophages, likely accelerate this process. Activated granulocytes sequestered in the lungs may cause acute cardiopulmonary complications. Neonates have a limited granulocyte pool in their bone marrow, which can be exhausted rapidly during overwhelming bacte-

rial sepsis. These infants may benefit from granulocyte transfusions or treatment with granulocyte colony-stimulating factor (G-CSF).

MEDICATIONS

Drug-induced neutropenia is a common and expected side effect of anticancer therapy. Many chemotherapeutic agents have a direct toxic effect on the early marrow stem cells. The severity and duration of the neutropenia depend on the particular medication, dosage, underlying disease, and state of nutrition and general health. These children should follow general supportive care guidelines for chronic neutropenia by taking prophylactic trimethoprim–sulfamethoxazole (to prevent *Pneumocystis carinii*) and oral Mycostatin as needed for thrush, adhering to vigorous mouth care, avoiding exposure to crowds and sick people, and receiving prophylactic varicella zoster immune globulin for varicella exposures.

Many other medications can induce neutropenia, including antibiotics (chloramphenicol, cephalosporins, penicillins, sulfonamides), anticonvulsants (phenytoin, valproic acid), anti-inflammatory agents, cardiovascular agents, tranquilizers, and hypoglycemic agents. The severity and duration of drug-induced neutropenia are variable. The underlying mechanism is not known, although studies with certain drugs have led to various hypotheses: immune mediated, a toxic effect of the drug or metabolites on the marrow stem cells, and toxic effects on the marrow microenvironment. After withdrawal of the drug, the marrow can repopulate with early myeloid forms within 3 to 4 days and appear morphologically normal by 1 to 2 weeks. The duration of neutropenia is likely related to the underlying mechanism; some chronic idiosyncratic drug reactions can last from months to years. Immune-mediated neutropenia usually resolves within 6 to 8 days of withdrawal of the offending agent.

Neonatal Alloimmune Neutropenia

Neonatal alloimmune neutropenia, analogous to Rh hemolytic anemia and neonatal alloimmune thrombocytopenia, can occur as a result of maternal sensitization to fetal neutrophil antigens during gestation. This results in the formation of immunoglobulin G antibodies that cross the placenta and destroy the infant's neutrophils. The infants usually recover within 3 to 6 weeks, but can develop fever and life-threatening infections within the first few days after birth. Treatment of these infections may include use of antibiotics, G-CSF, plasma exchange, and infusion of maternal neutrophils known to lack the antigen to which the antibody is directed.

ORGANOMEGALY

Organomegaly, in particular splenic enlargement from any cause, can cause sequestration of circulating neutrophils, resulting in neutropenia. Anemia and thrombocytopenia may also occur. Treatment of the underlying disease process often ameliorates the neutropenia.

DIAGNOSTIC APPROACH TO THE CHILD WITH NEUTROPENIA

Evaluation of the child with neutropenia begins with a thorough history and physical examination. Included should be the child's family history, medication list, recent illnesses, age, and ethnicity. On examination, attention should be paid to any phenotypic abnormalities, adenopathy, splenomegaly, evidence of a chronic or underlying disease, and meticulous evaluation of the skin and mucous membranes (oral and perirectal). The laboratory evaluation helps establish the severity and duration (using periodic blood counts) of the neutropenia. Patients with chronic neutropenia should have blood counts checked twice a week for 6 weeks to evaluate for cyclic neutropenia.

Additional studies include antineutrophil antibodies, assessment of cellular and serum immune status, and careful review of the peripheral smear for morphologic abnormalities of the white cells. Hematologic values, red cell indices, and platelet studies should also be done. A bone marrow aspirate and biopsy may be necessary to identify granulocyte precursors and to search for defects in myeloid maturation. In addition, the bone marrow aspirate and biopsy can be used to exclude hematologic malignancies, marrow infiltration, or fibrosis.

MANAGEMENT OF THE CHILD WITH NEUTROPENIA

The management of neutropenia depends on many factors, including the nature of the neutropenia (acute or chronic), its severity, and the association with immune defects, underlying illnesses, and malignancies (Fig. 13–1). Patients with acquired neutropenia arising from malignancy or chemotherapeutic drugs have a diminished inflammatory capability and are unusually susceptible to sepsis. Fever may be the earliest and only warning sign. Sepsis related to induced neutropenia remains a leading cause of mortality in these patients. Aggressive management of the febrile, neutropenic patient in the hospital has markedly reduced morbidity and mortality resulting from infection.

The **febrile neutropenic patient** warrants emergent medical assessment and initiation of therapy. The chronicity and severity of the neutropenia influence the type of infectious pathogen and severity of infection. In children with chronic benign neutropenia with fever, it is more likely that a viral pathogen is present; however, the child should be evaluated by a health care practitioner. The child with severe neutropenia (such as congenital neutropenia, or Kostmann's disease) may require hospital admission as a result of evidence of sepsis or need for broad-spectrum coverage with parenteral antibiotics.

The initial evaluation of the child with fever and neutropenia includes meticulous physical examination with particular attention to sites of occult

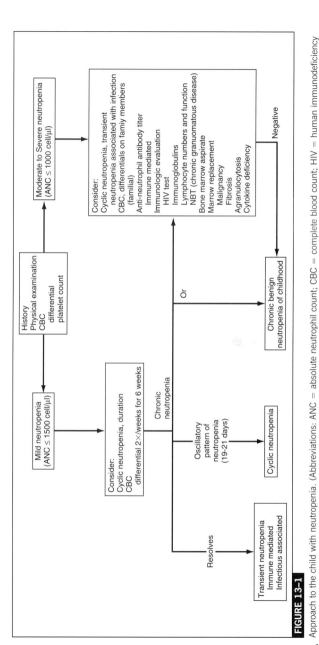

FIGURE 13-1

Approach to the child with neutropenia. (Abbreviations: ANC = absolute neutrophil count; CBC = complete blood count; HIV = human immunodeficiency virus; NBT = nitroblue tetrazolium.)

MANAGEMENT OF THE CHILD WITH NEUTROPENIA

infection (the oral cavity and perineum) a complete blood count with differential, blood culture, urinalysis and urine culture, chest radiograph if pulmonary symptoms are present, and cultures from sites of suspected infection, such as skin, throat, and stool. Blood cultures and complete blood counts with differentials should be obtained every 24 hours in the persistently febrile patient. Broad-spectrum antibiotics must be started immediately and provide coverage for gram-negative and gram-positive organisms. A combination of an aminoglycoside and a β-lactam antibiotic provides initial broad coverage and is synergistic for *Pseudomonas* species. The child who appears well and has a known history of chronic benign neutropenia may be treated with a β-lactam antibiotic, such as ceftriaxone, and be monitored as an outpatient. G-CSF may be indicated in some patients. If the child defervesces, the cultures remain negative, and the clinical course improves, the antibiotics can be discontinued after 72 hours depending on the degree of neutropenia and expected duration. For management of oncology patients with fever and neutropenia, see Chapter 19.

SUGGESTED READING

Dinauer MC. The phagocyte system and disorders of granulopoiesis and granulocyte function. In: Nathan DG, Orkin SH (eds), Nathan and Oski's Hematology of Infancy and Childhood, 5th ed. Philadelphia: WB Saunders, 1998, pp 889–967.

Hastings CA, Lubin BH. Blood. In: Rudolph AM, Kamei RK (eds), Rudolph's Fundamentals of Pediatrics, 2nd ed. Norwalk, CT: Appleton & Lange, 1998, pp 441–490.

Lanzowsky P. Manual of Pediatric Hematology and Oncology, 3rd ed. San Diego: Academic Press, 2000.

IMMUNE-MEDIATED THROMBOCYTOPENIA

The initial evaluation of thrombocytopenia requires confirmation of the platelet count on review of the peripheral smear, especially in the nonsymptomatic child. False values for platelet counts can result from aggregation of platelets in the syringe or collection tube, counting of small nonplatelet particles (fragmented red or white cells) by automated cell counters, and pseudothrombocytopenia caused by in vitro platelet agglutination by anticoagulant-dependent ethylenediaminetetra-acetic acid (EDTA) antibodies. Review of the blood film may show clumps of agglutinated platelets at the periphery of the slide. Thrombocytopenia is defined as a platelet count less than 100×10^9/L. The differential diagnosis of thrombocytopenia in children is shown in Table 14–1, and the approach to managing the child with thrombocytopenia is presented in Figures 14–1, 14–2, and 14–3.

The most common cause of destructive thrombocytopenia is immune-mediated platelet destruction. Shortened platelet survival can result from an immunoglobulin G antibody directed against a platelet membrane antigen, either an autoantigen or possibly a neoantigen resulting from infection with a microorganism or drug exposure. Immunoglobulin M antibodies and complement activation are less frequently found but can also be seen in childhood immune thrombocytopenic purpura (ITP).

IMMUNE THROMBOCYTOPENIC PURPURA

ITP is an acute, self-limited disease of isolated thrombocytopenia that usually occurs in children ages 2 to 4 years; it usually resolves within 6 months. When ITP occurs in the child younger than 1 year or over 10 years of age, the course is often chronic and associated with a generalized immune disorder. The otherwise healthy child presents with sudden onset of severe thrombocytopenia, manifest by petechiae, purpura, epistaxis, and, less frequently, hematuria and gastrointestinal hemorrhage. There may be a history of an antecedent viral illness within the past 1 to 3 weeks. Death from ITP is rare (<1%) and usually due to intracranial hemorrhage.

EVALUATION

Initial evaluation of the child with suspected ITP begins with a complete history and physical examination. Other than a possible antecedent illness and the acute onset of minor bleeding and bruising, the child is well. There is no hepatosplenomegaly or significant adenopathy (other than that seen with a mild viral illness). There should be no evidence of chronic disease, weight loss, fevers, or bone pain.

TABLE 14-1

DIFFERENTIAL DIAGNOSIS OF THROMBOCYTOPENIA

Destructive Thrombocytopenias

Immunologic
  ITP
  Drug induced
  Infection induced
  Post-transfusion purpura
  Autoimmune disease
  Post-transplant
  Hyperthyroidism
  Lymphoproliferative disorders
Nonimmunologic
  Microangiopathic disease
  Hemolytic anemia and thrombocytopenia
  Hemolytic–uremic syndrome
  Thrombotic thrombocytopenic purpura
Platelet Consumption/Destruction
  DIC
  Giant hemangiomas
  Cardiac (prosthetic heart valves, repair of intracardiac defects)
Neonatal Problems
  Pulmonary hypertension
  Polycythemia
  RDS/infection (viral, bacterial, protozoal, spirochetal)
  Sepsis/DIC
  Prematurity
  Meconium aspiration
  Giant hemangioma
  Neonatal alloimmune
  Neonatal autoimmune (maternal ITP)
  Erythroblastosis fetalis (Rh incompatibility)

Impaired Production

Congenital & Hereditary Disorders
  Thrombocytopenia–absent radii (TAR) syndrome
  Fanconi's anemia
  Bernard-Soulier syndrome
  Wiskott-Aldrich syndrome
  Glanzmann's thrombasthenia
  May-Hegglin anomaly
  Amegakaryocytosis (congenital)
  Rubella syndrome
Associated with Chromosomal Defect
  Trisomy 13 or 18
Metabolic disorders
  Marrow infiltration: malignancies, storage disease, myelofibrosis
Acquired processes
  Aplastic anemia
  Drug induced
  Severe iron deficiency

Table continued on opposite page

TABLE 14–1

DIFFERENTIAL DIAGNOSIS OF THROMBOCYTOPENIA *Continued*

Sequestration

Hypersplenism (portal hypertension, neoplastic, infectious, glycogen storage disease, cyanotic heart disease)

Hypothermia

Abbreviations: ITP = immune thrombocytopenic purpura; DIC = disseminated intravascular coagulation; RDS = respiratory distress syndrome.

Review of the peripheral blood smear confirms a low platelet count, and the few remaining platelets typically are large. If platelet size is determined by an automated cell counter, it is elevated, consistent with young platelet age and rapid platelet destruction. The erythrocyte and leukocyte counts are normal and there is no evidence of hemolysis or microangiopathic disease. Lymphocyte morphology may reflect a recent viral infection. If any findings suggest another diagnosis, consideration should be given to performing a bone marrow aspiration.

14

IMMUNE THROMBOCYTOPENIC PURPURA

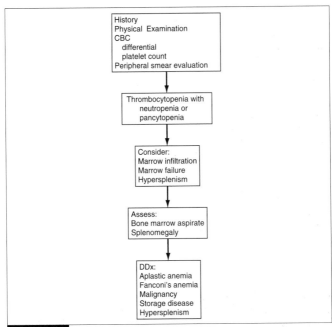

FIGURE 14–1

Approach to the child with thrombocytopenia with neutropenia or pancytopenia. (Abbreviations: CBC = complete blood count; DDx = differential diagnosis.)

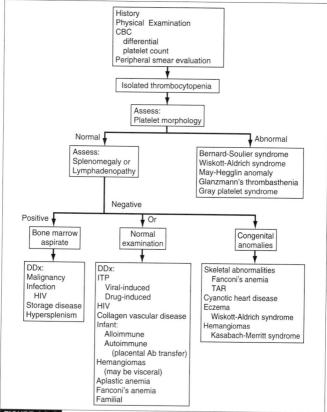

FIGURE 14-2

Approach to the child with isolated thrombocytopenia. (Abbreviations: CBC = complete blood count; DDx = differential diagnosis; HIV = human immunodeficiency virus; ITP = immune thrombocytopenic purpura; Ab = antibody; TAR = thrombocytopenia–absent radii.) *(From Hastings CA, Lubin BH. Blood. In: Rudolph AM, Kamei RK [eds], Rudolph's Fundamentals of Pediatrics, 2nd ed. Norwalk, CT: Appleton & Lange, 1998, pp 441–490; reprinted with permission.)*

The presence of immature megakaryocytes in normal or increased numbers in the marrow with normal erythroid and myeloid lineages confirms that the thrombocytopenia is due to increased peripheral destruction and supports the diagnosis of ITP.

By convention, a bone marrow aspirate is done on individuals with suspected ITP only if steroids are to be part of the treatment plan, because of the small possibility that the thrombocytopenia may actually be an early manifestation of leukemia.

A careful **drug history** should be obtained to identify agents that can interfere with platelet function, with particular attention to heparin, aspirin, aspirin-containing cold medications, nonsteroidal anti-inflammatory drugs, and seizure medications. Agents that alter platelet function must be avoided. Human immunodeficiency virus (HIV) infection should be considered when evaluating a patient with isolated thrombocytopenia, because this may be a first manifestation of infection in children. Screen for risk factors and test for HIV, if appropriate.

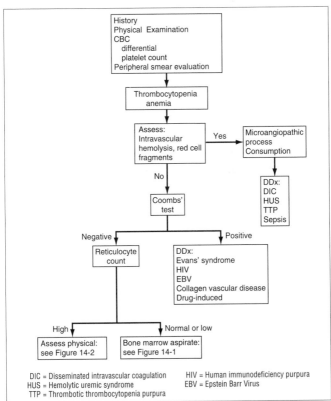

IMMUNE THROMBOCYTOPENIC PURPURA

FIGURE 14–3

Approach to the child with thrombocytopenia and anemia. (Abbreviations: CBC = complete blood count; DDx = differential diagnosis; HIV = human immunodeficiency virus; EBV = Epstein-Barr virus; DIC = disseminated intravascular coagulation; HUS = hemolytic–uremic syndrome; TTP = thrombotic thrombocytopenic purpura.)

The **physical examination** should include particular attention to the presence of skeletal anomalies, as can be seen in thrombocytopenia–absent radii syndrome and Fanconi's anemia (short stature, radial limb dysplasia), diseases that can present with thrombocytopenia. Evidence of microangiopathic disease on the smear, fever, and central nervous system symptoms can be seen in thrombotic thrombocytopenic purpura and hemolytic–uremic syndrome. Small platelets are seen in Wiskott-Aldrich syndrome, an X-linked disorder characterized by immunologic abnormalities, eczema, and recurrent infections. Patients with aplastic anemia may present initially with thrombocytopenia before progressing to pancytopenia.

A search for platelet antibodies may be conducted on some patients with acute thrombocytopenia. Assays for direct antibody measurement involve determining the antibodies coating the platelets, whereas indirect assays measure antiplatelet immunoglobulin in the plasma.

TREATMENT

Because the natural history of acute ITP is to resolve gradually and completely, the decision regarding whether to treat the patient becomes controversial. Many patients who have been observed carefully without pharmacologic intervention have done well. All patients and families should be counseled regarding rough play, contact sports and the use of protective gear (helmets), and use of car seats and seat belts. Intramuscular injections should be withheld until platelet counts increase. Specific medications that interfere with platelet function should not be given.

For children with platelet counts below 20×10^9/L, extensive oral or nasal mucosal hemorrhage, retinal petechiae, or severe hemorrhage, therapy with **intravenous immune globulin** (IVIG) is usually given as the first-line therapy. Treatment with IVIG, 0.8 to 1 g/kg over 4 to 6 hours, is often therapeutic. This treatment may need to be repeated two to three times (minimum 24 hours apart) for a total dose of 2 to 3 g/kg; doses should be given at least 24 hours apart. A rise in the platelet count is usually seen within 24 to 72 hours and peaks at approximately 9 days. IVIG is thought to saturate the Fc receptors on the reticuloendothelial cells and thereby decrease the clearance of opsonized platelets. Side effects of IVIG are usually immediate and related to the rate of infusion and include nausea, lightheadedness, and headache. These symptoms can be alleviated with further doses by slowing the rate of infusion. Fever may also occur, and premedication with acetaminophen before the infusion is advisable.

Corticosteroids have also been used in the medical management of ITP. Response is slightly slower than with IVIG. The usual steroid prescribed is prednisone, 1 to 2 mg/kg/day for 10 to 20 days, tapering the dosage over 2 weeks. Many patients respond to this treatment, but side effects may occur with repeated treatment or chronic use. An alternative to oral ste-

roids has been pulsed high-dose infusion of intravenous methylprednisolone. Some patients become thrombocytopenic again after therapy and require retreatment. A recurrence may be managed safely by observation
and restriction of activity and medications, or with intermittent IVIG or
pulsed steroids.

If the patient has evidence of central nervous system hemorrhage and remains severely thrombocytopenic and unresponsive to IVIG and steroids, an
emergency splenectomy should be considered. Continuous infusion of
platelets is advised to control bleeding, and plasmapheresis should be considered, although the response is very limited.

CHRONIC IDIOPATHIC THROMBOCYTOPENIC PURPURA

Approximately 10% to 20% of children with acute ITP develop chronic, persistent thrombocytopenia beyond 6 months. The child with chronic ITP
may have an associated autoimmune disease or immunodeficiency state.
Many patents with chronic ITP may not need treatment because the platelet
count is often above 20×10^9/L. IVIG may still provide effective therapy in
chronic ITP. Spontaneous remission can occur in these patients, and
some remissions have been reported 2 years after the original diagnosis.
Platelet count alone does not correlate with the risk of hemorrhage because
platelets are large and, as a consequence, not be picked up in the automated counters and additionally have a greater than normal procoagulant
activity.

In the rare patient with chronic, refractory ITP who has clinical hemorrhage or cannot tolerate the living restrictions imposed by the thrombocytopenia, splenectomy should be considered. Up to 60% to 85% of patients
respond to splenectomy; however, recurrence of ITP may occur as a
result of immune-mediated platelet destruction in other organs. Infusion of
RhoGAM (anti-Rh immune globulin) in nonsplenectomized Rh-positive
individuals has been used with some success in selected patients requiring
therapy. Vinca alkaloids (vincristine and vinblastine), danazol (a nonviril-
izing androgen), and immunosuppressive agents such as azathioprine and
cyclophosphamide have also been used with some success. Ascorbic
acid, cyclosporine, and interferon alfa-2b are other agents that have been
investigated for use in chronic ITP.

NEONATAL ALLOIMMUNE THROMBOCYTOPENIA

Neonatal alloimmune thrombocytopenia (NATP) is a rare syndrome that occurs in approximately 1 in 5000 newborns. The pathophysiology is similar to that of Rh disease. Immunization against the platelet alloantigens can
occur through either pregnancy or transfusion, and lead to severe thrombocytopenia in the fetal–newborn period, with a high risk of fatal hemorrhage. Several platelet antigens (PL^A) have been implicated, but the greatest
number of cases can be related to PL^{A1} incompatibility. PL^{A1} is a platelet
antigen that resides on the glycoprotein IIb/IIIa complex (the complex

14

NEONATAL ALLOIMMUNE THROMBOCYTOPENIA

responsible for the fibrinogen receptor activity of platelets and important in aggregation and platelet plug information). Development of anti-PL^{A1} antibodies therefore not only can decrease platelet number, but also can interfere with normal platelet aggregation, resulting in a qualitative defect in the platelets in addition to thrombocytopenia. This likely explains the high incidence of serious bleeding in these infants after birth or in utero as compared with infants born to mothers with ITP who have antibodies that are not directed against PL^{A1}.

PRESENTATION

The typical presentation of the affected infant with NATP is an otherwise healthy newborn, without perinatal complications and with a normal maternal hematologic history, who develops petechiae, purpura, and thrombocytopenia. For a mother with a previous low platelet count, the differential diagnosis includes maternal autoimmune or drug-dependent thrombocytopenia, infection, and pre-eclampsia. The infant who has birth asphyxia, infection, or congenital bone marrow hypoplasia, or who is premature, can also be thrombocytopenic. The presence of hepatosplenomegaly, intrauterine growth retardation, or intracranial calcifications with thrombocytopenia suggests a congenital viral infection. However, it is also important to exclude alloimmune thrombocytopenia by appropriate immunologic testing in these infants because there is a potential recurrence of this complication in future pregnancies.

In 50% of cases of NATP, first-born offspring are affected (unlike Rh incompatibility, which occurs primarily at the time of delivery), suggesting that antigenic exposure occurs early in pregnancy. This type of neonatal thrombocytopenia accounts for most cases of fetal morbidity and mortality. Bleeding manifestations tend to be more severe than in an infant with passive transfer of platelet antibody from the mother (maternal ITP).

Evidence of intrauterine intracranial hemorrhage can be seen on ultrasound. Even a platelet count less than 50×10^9/L warrants concern, especially if the infant was born by vaginal delivery.

Complications of early central nervous system hemorrhage include hydrocephalus, porencephaly, seizures, and fetal loss. Early jaundice occurs in 20% of cases as a result of resolution of intracranial or intraorgan hemorrhage. The thrombocytopenia is transient, lasting up to 3 to 6 weeks after delivery. An early platelet alloantigen evaluation of the newborn and parents is important, both to offer the affected infant treatment and to prevent such devastating complications with future pregnancies. Platelet typing should be done on the mother and father, looking for antigens responsible for alloimmunization in particular, as well as other platelet antigens frequently involved in alloimmune thrombocytopenia. The serum from the mother should be screened for anti-platelet antibodies. Studies should be done with maternal, and paternal or neonatal platelets to screen for platelet antigens. However, the infant's platelet count may be too low to make this assessment.

TREATMENT AND PREVENTION

Several treatment options are available for the infant with neonatal alloimmunization. Transfusion with antigen-negative platelets has been the mainstay of treatment. Because PL^{A1} antigen–negative platelets are present in
only 2% of the population, the most readily available source of platelets
is the mother. Random platelets may provide a transient increase, lasting
1 to 2 days, and should be used in cases of serious hemorrhage while
antigen-negative platelets are being obtained and prepared. An excellent alternative treatment is the administration of IVIG. The recommended dose
is 1 g/kg/24 hours for 1 to 2 doses until the platelet count is over $50 \times
10^9$/L. Platelet transfusion may still be necessary with IVIG if immediate
correction of the thrombocytopenia is needed. Corticosteroids can be effective in reducing platelet destruction and increasing vascular integrity. Frequent head ultrasounds should be done while the child remains severely thrombocytopenic ($<50 \times 10^9$/L).

A mother who has one child with NATP is at high risk for having subsequent infants with the same disease. The severity of antenatal and perinatal
hemorrhage is also increased. Maternal antiplatelet titers cannot be used
to predict affected fetuses accurately. Fetal cord blood samples should be
obtained periodically for determination of the platelet count starting at about
20 weeks of gestation, with ultrasound monitoring for hemorrhage. Studies done on mothers treated with IVIG 1 g/kg/week from midgestation until
near term have shown increases in fetal platelet count in the majority of
cases; this approach should be considered. Delivery should be planned near
term with an elective cesarean section or planned induced vaginal delivery
after documented increase in fetal platelet count following administration
of maternal IVIG. Antigen-negative platelets should be obtained and prepared prior to delivery in the event of extreme thrombocytopenia or hemorrhage. The mother can be platelet-pheresed prior to delivery to obtain
PL^{A1}-negative platelets. The infant's platelet count should be checked at
birth and every 6 to 12 hours for 1 to 2 days, then daily, and be kept at or
above 20×10^9/L.

DRUG-INDUCED THROMBOCYTOPENIA

In addition to immune-mediated mechanisms for thrombocytopenia
induced by drugs, many bone marrow–suppressive agents used in
chemotherapy cause thrombocytopenia, usually in the face of pancytopenia. Management is usually with platelet transfusion, to prevent or
treat bleeding. The bone marrow effects of these agents define their dose-
limiting toxicities, and thrombocytopenia is a common and anticipated
problem. These patients usually respond well to platelet transfusion but
can become refractory because of the underlying illness, organomegaly
and sequestration, development of alloimmunization, sepsis, and other
medications.

14

DRUG-INDUCED THROMBOCYTOPENIA

SUGGESTED READING

Beardsley DS. Platelet abnormalities in infancy and childhood. In: Nathan DG, Orkin SH (eds), Nathan and Oski's Hematology of Infancy and Childhood, 5th ed. Philadelphia: WB Saunders, 1998, pp 1585–1630.

Hastings CA, Lubin BH. Blood. In: Rudolph AM, Kamei RK (eds), Rudolph's Fundamentals of Pediatrics, 2nd ed. Norwalk, CT: Appleton & Lange, 1998, pp 441–490.

Lankowsky P. Manual of Pediatric Hematology and Oncology, 3rd ed. San Diego: Academic Press, 2000.

NON–IMMUNE-MEDIATED THROMBOCYTOPENIA

INCREASED PLATELET CONSUMPTION

Several non–immune-mediated processes involve increased platelet consumption. Generalized platelet activation with trapping of microaggregates in the small vasculature contributes to the microangiopathic hemolytic anemia occurring in the hemolytic–uremic syndrome and thrombotic thrombocytopenic purpura. Increased utilization of the platelets may occur in active bleeding or infection.

15

DISSEMINATED INTRAVASCULAR COAGULATION

In disseminated intravascular coagulation (DIC), there is an imbalance between intravascular thrombosis and fibrinolysis, with increased platelet consumption, depletion of plasma clotting factors, and formation of fibrin. DIC can be initiated by many events, including sepsis cause by bacteria, viruses, or fungi; malignancy, particularly acute promyelocytic leukemia and neuroblastoma; hemolytic transfusion reactions; and trauma. Therapy is aimed at the underlying etiologic process; supportive care consists of platelet transfusion to maintain platelet counts over 50 to 100×10^9/L and plasma protein replenishment (cryoprecipitate, fresh frozen plasma to correct coagulopathies and maintain fibrinogen greater than 100 mg/dl).

THE SICK NEWBORN

Thrombocytopenia can occur in the sick newborn for many reasons, most commonly with infection, prematurity, asphyxia, respiratory distress syndrome, pulmonary hypertension, or meconium aspiration. These infants appear to have normal to increased platelet production, but have a decreased platelet life span for reasons that are unclear. Thrombocytopenia is a frequent occurrence in congenital cyanotic heart disease associated with compensatory polycythemia. Therapeutic phlebotomy may lessen the thrombocytopenia.

KASABACH-MERRITT SYNDROME

The association of thrombocytopenia and giant hemangiomas occurs in the infant with Kasabach-Merritt syndrome. The hemangiomas may be multiple and may involve only viscera. Therefore, in an infant with unexplained thrombocytopenia, imaging studies should be done to look for a vascular anomaly. Hemangiomas are proliferative lesions that grow rapidly for several months and then regress spontaneously. Platelet thrombi may develop in these lesions, and platelet life span may be decreased. These infants may also have a consumptive coagulopathy with low fibrinogen levels and elevated concentrations of fibrin degradation products. The lesions are prone to necrosis and infection. A particular hemangioma's size or location cannot predict whether it will lead to platelet trapping and thrombocytopenia.

117

These infants should be managed by close observation and hematologic monitoring, waiting for regression to occur. However, the lesions may become large enough to compromise the infant (impinge on the airway or vital organs, leading to compartment syndrome), resulting in serious illness or death. Corticosteroid treatment may be beneficial at a dose of 1 to 2 mg/kg/day of prednisone until regression of the lesion or normalization of the platelet count occurs, with subsequent tapering. Interferon alfa-2a has been reported to be beneficial in correcting the platelet count and shrinking the lesion; it has been given in doses of 1 to 3 million U/m^2/day. This treatment may be used alone or in combination with steroids and is under further investigation. Supportive transfusion therapy may be necessary when the infant is at risk of hemorrhage; platelet transfusions are given daily, in addition to plasma and cryoprecipitate if there is fibrinogen consumption. Antiplatelet medications (aspirin and dipyridamole) have been used in the past to interfere with platelet trapping within the hemangioma, but they carry the risk of causing platelet dysfunction in addition to the thrombocytopenia.

DECREASED PLATELET PRODUCTION

Congenital amegakaryocytic thrombocytopenia, a rare cause of neonatal thrombocytopenia, may be caused by a congenital viral infection or an inherited disorder, or be idiopathic. Cytomegalovirus, rubella, and human immunodeficiency virus all have been associated with hypoproductive thrombocytopenia. Neutropenia and anemia are often associated findings. The **thrombocytopenia–absent radii syndrome** is an autosomal recessive disorder with variable thrombocytopenia despite normal erythroid and myeloid lineages. Many patients are transfusion dependent, but may experience a spontaneous increase in megakaryocytopoiesis after 1 year of age. **Fanconi's anemia** is another inherited disorder with both skeletal anomalies and hypoproductive thrombocytopenia, although other cell lines are affected. The cytopenia begins in early to late childhood and is associated with chromosomal instability. Infants with hypoproductive states, including **Wiskott-Aldrich syndrome**, viral infection, or an inherited giant platelet syndrome such as the **May-Hegglin anomaly** or **Bernard-Soulier syndrome**, may have other reasons for isolated thrombocytopenia. Evaluation of the peripheral smear and possibly a bone marrow aspirate help confirm the diagnosis.

SUGGESTED READING

Beardsley DS. Platelet abnormalities in infancy and childhood. In: Nathan DG, Orkin SH (eds), Nathan and Oski's Hematology of Infancy and Childhood 5th ed. Philadelphia: WB Saunders, 1998, pp 1585–1630.

Lanzkowsky P. Manual of Pediatric Hematology and Oncology, 3rd ed. San Diego: Academic Press, 2000.

INITIAL EVALUATION OF THE CHILD WITH A SUSPECTED MALIGNANCY

Each year approximately 6500 children under age 15 years are diagnosed with cancer in the United States. Though cancer remains the second leading cause of death in children, after accidents, survival continues to steadily increase. More than 65% of children diagnosed with cancer are now expected to be cured of their disease. Cancer is a devastating diagnosis. The initial approach to the child and the family must be with a heightened sensitivity of this family tragedy.

The diagnosis of cancer in a child starts with a thorough history and physical examination. The history is the first step in the diagnostic process, with the chief complaint being the most important clue. The most common chief complaints and their associated malignancies are listed in Table 16-1. Most of the symptoms of childhood cancer are due to either a mass, its effect on the surrounding tissues, invasion of the marrow, or secretion of a substance by the tumor that disturbs normal function. A careful family history should be elicited and should include familial cancers and genetic diseases, such as Down syndrome, neurofibromatosis, and autoimmune diseases. Environmental and genetic factors have been associated with the development of malignancy, though the latter probably play a more significant role in pediatric cancer. The most common signs and symptoms of pediatric cancer are listed in Table 16-2.

Treatment of a malignancy can only start after accurate diagnosis and staging. This process will likely involve radiographic assessment and pathologic diagnosis (bone marrow aspirate in hematologic malignancies).

PRESENTATION

HEADACHE
Headache is one of the most common symptoms of cancer in the pediatric population. Although few headaches are caused by intracranial masses, primary brain tumors or metastasis must be ruled out when dealing with a patient with repeated headaches. Increased intracranial pressure is a common occurrence in pediatric brain tumors and is related to location. Radiographic evaluation with computed tomography (CT) (Table 16-3) or magnetic resonance imaging (MRI) is recommended in children with symptoms suggestive of a brain tumor: recurrent morning headache, headache that awakens the child, intense incapacitating headache, and changes in the quality, frequency, and pattern of the headaches. A thorough neurologic examination should precede radiographic imaging.

TABLE 16–1

COMMON CHIEF COMPLAINTS GIVEN BY PARENTS THAT SUGGEST A PEDIATRIC CANCER

CHIEF COMPLAINT	SUGGESTED CANCER
Chronic drainage from ear	Langerhans' cell histiocytosis
Recurrent fever with bone pain	Leukemia, Ewing's sarcoma, neuroblastoma
Morning headache with vomiting	Brain tumor
Lump in neck that does not respond to antibiotics	Hodgkin's or non-Hodgkin's lymphomas, leukemia
White dot in eye	Retinoblastoma
Swollen face and neck	Non-Hodgkin's lymphoma, leukemia
Mass in abdomen	Wilms' tumor, neuroblastoma, hepatoma
Paleness and fatigue	Leukemia, lymphoma
Limping	Osteosarcoma, other bone tumors, leukemia
Bone pain	Leukemia, Ewing's sarcoma, neuroblastoma
Bleeding from vagina	Yolk sac tumor, rhabdomyosarcoma
Weight loss	Hodgkin's lymphoma
Mass in extremity	Rhabdomyosarcoma, bone tumors

LYMPHADENOPATHY

Lymphadenopathy is a common finding on exam in association with malignancies and infection. A lymph node is considered enlarged if it is larger than 10 mm, with the exception of epitrochlear nodes, for which 5 mm is considered abnormal, and inguinal nodes, which are not considered abnormal unless the size is 15 mm or greater. Most children have shotty ade-

TABLE 16–2

PRESENTING SIGNS AND SYMPTOMS OF SOME COMMON PEDIATRIC CANCERS AND THEIR DIFFERENTIAL DIAGNOSES

PRESENTING SIGNS OR SYMPTOMS	COMMON DIAGNOSES (NONMALIGNANT CONDITIONS)	CANCER
Headache, morning vomiting	Migraine, sinusitis	Brain tumor
Lymphadenopathy	Infection	Lymphoma, leukemia
Bone pain	Infection, trauma	Bone tumor, leukemia
Abdominal mass	Constipation, kidney cyst, full bladder	Wilms' tumor, neuroblastoma
Mediastinal mass	Infection, cysts	Lymphomas
Pancytopenia	Infection	Leukemia
Bleeding	Coagulation disorders, platelet disorders, ITP	Leukemia, neuroblastoma
Back pain	Trauma	Leukemia, lymphoma, CNS tumor or extension of abdominal tumor into spinal cord

Abbreviations: ITP = immune thrombocytopenic purpura; CNS = central nervous system.

TABLE 16-3

CONDITIONS SUGGESTING NEED FOR COMPUTED TOMOGRAPHY IN CHILDREN WITH HEADACHE

Presence or onset of neurologic abnormality

Ocular findings such as papilledema, decreased visual acuity, or loss of vision

Vomiting that is persistent, increasing in frequency, or preceded by recurrent headaches

Change in character of headache, such as increased severity and frequency

Recurrent morning headaches or headaches that repeatedly awaken child from sleep

Short stature or deceleration of linear growth

Diabetes insipidus

Age 3 years or less

Neurofibromatosis

History of acute lymphoblastic leukemia with irradiation of central nervous system

nopathy in the cervical, posterior auricular, and inguinal areas. Adenopathy in the supraclavicular, axillary, or epitrochlear areas is definitely abnormal. Adenopathy that persists longer than 6 weeks should arouse concern for malignancy. Asymmetric lymphadenopathy is a worrisome clue. Lymphadenopathy associated with a viral infection usually resolves spontaneously in 2 to 6 weeks. Leukemia typically presents with generalized lymphadenopathy. Localized adenopathy may be infectious in origin; etiologies include bacterial (typically *Staphylococcus aureus* or β-hemolytic streptococcal species), human immunodeficiency virus, Epstein-Barr virus, cat-scratch disease, toxoplasmosis, cytomegalovirus (CMV), and nontuberculous mycobacteria. Localized cervical adenitis with inflammation and fever should be treated with antibiotics. Obtain a complete blood count (CBC) with a differential and assess the peripheral blood smear for possible abnormal cells (atypical lymphocytes in viral infection; lymphoblasts in malignancy; toxic granulocytes in bacterial infections).

If a lymph node is increasing in size, it should be biopsied. Children with mildly enlarged nodes should be monitored with frequent exams; when increase is not associated with malignancy, most of these nodes will revert to normal size. Malignant nodes are generally hard and nontender. Nodes secondary to infection or inflammation tend to feel more rubbery, often are tender, and have an overlying erythema.

If there is no response to antibiotics and/or the node is 3 cm in size, a further work-up should continue and include purified protein derivative (for tuberculosis), chest radiograph, repeat CBC with differential, chemistries including lactate dehydrogenase (LDH) and uric acid, and serologies as indicated by history and examination. A biopsy should be done on enlarging or persistently large nodes or if adenopathy is also seen on chest radiograph.

BONE PAIN

Bone pain associated with cancer is usually due to bone, nerve, or marrow involvement. Leukemia commonly presents with bone pain. Bone pain can also be a presenting symptom in patients with bone tumors, osteogenic sarcoma, or Ewing's sarcoma. Arthritis can be a presenting symptom in acute leukemia, and, in association with anemia or leukopenia, should prompt examination of the bone marrow. Localized bone pain warrants radiographic evaluation for assessment of a lesion or leukemic changes.

PANCYTOPENIA

Anemia, leukopenia, and thrombocytopenia can occur alone (though rarely) or in combination as a common presenting sign in acute leukemia. The pancytopenia is largely the result of replacement of the marrow by a malignant population of cells. Anemia is frequently characterized as one of chronic disease (normochromic, low reticulocyte count) though may be secondary to hemorrhage within a mass, either chronic or acute. Except with marrow involvement, leukopenia and thrombocytopenia are rarely associated with extramedullary malignancies. Disseminated intravascular coagulation (DIC) can be seen with neuroblastoma, rhabdomyosarcoma, and some forms of acute myelogenous leukemia (AML) (promyelocytic).

HYPERLEUKOCYTOSIS

Hyperleukocytosis is commonly seen with acute and chronic leukemias of childhood and is defined as a white cell count greater than $100,000/\mu l$. Elevated white cell counts ($>50,000/\mu l$) can be seen in septicemia and leukemoid reactions. Leukocytosis due to a markedly elevated eosinophil count can be seen in parasitic infections. Evaluation of the peripheral blood smear can help distinguish acute leukemia (blasts), chronic leukemia (myeloid-lineage cells in all phases of differentiation, may include early blasts), and a possible leukemoid reaction. Morphologic features of blast cells include abnormally large size, though many lymphoblasts may be the same size as lymphocytes; high nuclear:cytoplasmic ratio; presence of nucleoli; and unusual chromatin structure. Auer rods (red, sticklike structures in the cytoplasm) are pathognomonic for some forms of AML. Blasts are usually seen in association with thrombocytopenia and anemia.

EVALUATION OF THE CHILD WITH SUSPECTED LEUKEMIA

The work-up of a child with suspected leukemia includes a meticulous physical examination and careful history. The child should be assessed quickly for life-threatening situations such as severe anemia, thrombocytopenia, DIC, infection, compression of vital organs, hyperleukocytosis, and metabolic derangements.

LABORATORY STUDIES

1. CBC with manual differential, reticulocyte count, examination of peripheral blood smear for abnormal cells (blasts)

2. Electrolytes, blood urea nitrogen (BUN), creatinine, uric acid, LDH
3. Serum glutamate oxaloacetate transaminase, serum glutamate pyruvate transaminase, alkaline phosphatase, total bilirubin, magnesium, calcium, phosphorus
4. Serologies: varicella; CMV; herpes; hepatitis A, B, and C (obtain prior to start of therapy)
5. Quantitative immunoglobulins
6. Coagulation studies: prothrombin time/International Normalized Ratio, activated partial thromboplastin time, fibrin degradation products or D-dimers, fibrinogen
7. Type and cross for packed red blood cells if necessary
8. If febrile or ill-appearing: blood culture, urine culture

RADIOGRAPHIC STUDIES

1. Chest radiograph (assess for mediastinal mass)
2. Plain bone films of sites of bone pain (assess for pathologic fractures)

DIAGNOSTIC STUDIES

1. Bone marrow aspiration
   a. Specimens for morphology, immunophenotyping, karyotype
   b. Extra "pulls" as per protocol for biologic studies (Children's Oncology Group or local institutional studies)
   c. For "dry" taps, bone marrow biopsy for diagnostic studies
2. Lumbar puncture (platelet count >30 to 50×10^9/L)
   a. Cytology, chamber count (white cells, red cells, protein, glucose), cerebrospinal fluid culture if patient is febrile
   b. Initial procedure done by the pediatric oncology attending or fellow, after careful evaluation for elevated intracranial pressure

INITIAL MANAGEMENT (see Chapters 20 and 21)

1. Assess for emergent situations (metabolic abnormalities, tumor lysis syndrome, cardiovascular or respiratory compromise).
2. Obtain venous access; initiate hydration with two times maintenance fluids with alkalinization (5% dextrose in water + 40 mEq/L sodium bicarbonate, no K^+ in intravenous fluids).
3. Give allopurinol PO q8h or urate oxidase IV (if available) if labs show evidence of hyperuricemia or tumor lysis.
4. Obtain lysis labs q6h (electrolytes, calcium, uric acid, BUN, LDH, creatinine, phosphorus). Monitor CBC, other labs as indicated.
5. Transfuse (if possible, after all labs obtained) as indicated:
   a. PRBCs if the patient is hemodynamically unstable, evidence of congestive heart failure or bleeding
   b. Platelets if the platelet count is less than 30 to 50×10^9/L (prepare for lumbar puncture, placement of central line)

    c. PRBCs if the hemoglobin is less than 8 g/dl (prepare for induction therapy)

    d. Use caution when transfusing a child with hyperleukocytosis. Transfuse only if hemodynamically unstable and do not exceed a Hgb of 10 g/dl. Platelets may be given safely. See Chapter 20.

    e. **All initial blood products should be CMV negative (per institutional policy), irradiated, and leukocyte depleted.**

6. Provide psychological support of family (keep them informed).
7. Obtain surgical consult for possible placement of central venous catheter.
8. For fever or suspected infection, start antibiotics after cultures are obtained: broad-spectrum antibiotics per institutional practice (suggested: tobramycin 7.5 mg/kg/day divided q8h and ceftazidime 100 mg/kg/day divided q8h [assume all patients are functionally neutropenic]).
9. Review open Children's Oncology Group or local institutional protocols for eligibility.

EVALUATION OF THE CHILD WITH AN ABDOMINAL MASS

A malignant solid tumor should be suspected in a child with a palpable abdominal mass. Other etiologies include impacted stool, abdominal aorta, distended bladder, or hydronephrotic kidneys.

The **age** of the child can provide a clue to diagnosis. In the newborn, an abdominal mass is most likely to be renal in origin. The most common malignant tumors are **neuroblastoma** and **Wilms' tumor**. In older patients, the mass may be related to leukemia or lymphoma with enlargement of the spleen and liver.

The **history** can help determine if the symptoms are related to the mass. A good genitourinary history would be important in a suspected renal mass. Historical points may lead to suspicion of catecholamine production, such as flushing, palpitations, diarrhea, and sweating (very rare). Constitutional symptoms such as failure to thrive and fever should lead one to suspect a disseminated process, such as neuroblastoma.

The complete **examination** should include particular attention to the skin, extremities (bone pain), neurologic exam (Horner's syndrome, spinal cord compression), presence of organomegaly, and measurement of abdominal girth. Care should be taken to palpate the mass gently and limit the number of examiners. A rectal exam is a necessary part of the evaluation, and a pelvic exam with bimanual exam should be done in the older adolescent female.

DIAGNOSTIC IMAGING STUDIES

Diagnostic imaging studies include the following:

1. Flat plate of the abdomen with anteroposterior and lateral views
2. Chest radiograph: assess for metastases (Wilms', germ cell tumors, intrathoracic/intraspinal component of neuroblastoma)

3. Abdominal ultrasound
4. Abdominal CT scan: include chest and pelvis to assess for extent of disease and possible metastases
5. Bone scan and/or skeletal survey in suspected neuroblastoma, rhabdomyosarcoma, clear cell or rhabdoid tumor of the kidney
6. MRI of spine in tumors with neurologic impairment or radiographic suggestion of spinal invasion

LABORATORY STUDIES

1. CBC with differential, reticulocyte count (bleeding into mass may cause anemia, iron deficiency; tumor may involve the bone marrow and cause pancytopenia), review of peripheral smear
2. Electrolytes, calcium, phosphorus, uric acid, LDH, BUN, creatinine, liver transaminases
3. Urinalysis
4. Urine for catecholamines (vanillylmandelic acid, homovanillic acid)
5. Bone marrow aspirates/biopsies, if neuroblastoma suspected or confirmed

SURGICAL EVALUATION

A surgical evaluation should be obtained and the decision made regarding whether to obtain a biopsy, perform a resection of the mass, or both. Surgical staging is done by assessing possible tumor spillage, tumor margins, nodal involvement, and presence of locally invasive or distant disease (see Chapters 24 and 25).

SUGGESTED READING

Steuber CP, Nesbit ME. Clinical assessment and differential diagnosis of the child with suspected cancer. In: Pizzo PA, Poplack DG (eds), Principles and Practice of Pediatric Oncology, 3rd ed. Philadelphia: Lippincott–Raven, 1997, pp 129–140.

16

EVALUATION OF THE CHILD WITH AN ABDOMINAL MASS

SUPPORTIVE CARE OF THE CHILD WITH CANCER

INFECTION PROPHYLAXIS

Children receiving chemotherapy for treatment of their malignancies are susceptible to acquiring infection from bacterial, viral, fungal, and protozoal organisms. They are chronically myelosuppressed, and at times severely myelosuppressed, as a direct result of the chemotherapy, and have an increased exposure to nosocomial organisms. Many of these children have central venous catheters and may intermittently have mucosal breakdown secondary to chemotherapy, two situations that interrupt the integrity of the physical defense barriers. Hyponutrition also plays a significant role in host susceptibility. Certain standards of care are indicated to minimize the risk of acquiring infection in these children. Infection prophylaxis has been the cornerstone of supportive care in children with malignancies, decreasing morbidity and mortality from infection.

GENERAL MEASURES

General measures for the prevention of infection include avoidance of crowded environments, wearing a mask in public when severely neutropenic, and careful hand washing (by the patient and all those who have direct contact). Good nutrition and proper dental hygiene cannot be overemphasized. Oral hygiene should include daily brushing (with a soft brush) and use of chlorhexidine mouth rise (**Peridex**), or washing mouth with a mild sodium bicarbonate solution (1/2 teaspoon baking soda per cup of water). Cleanliness of the perirectal area is important, especially in the neutropenic state. Constipation should be avoided with age-appropriate diet, and, if necessary, a stool softener (e.g., docusate sodium). No rectal suppositories should be given and no rectal temperatures taken to avoid the possibility of a mucosal tear and entrance of enteric organisms.

BACTERIAL PROPHYLAXIS

Bacterial prophylaxis is indicated in immune-suppressed children to reduce the risk of acquiring *Pneumocystis carinii* pneumonia (PCP). Patients receiving chemotherapy have a higher incidence of PCP. Prophylactic trimethoprim–sulfamethoxazole (TMP-SMX) (5 mg/kg/day in 2 divided doses, 2 to 3 successive days a week) can effectively reduce this risk. Some evidence indicates that this regimen also provides good general antibacterial prophylaxis. For patients with allergy or intolerance to TMP-SMX, pentamidine or dapsone may be given. The dose of pentamidine is 4 mg/kg/dose IV diluted in 50 to 250 ml 5% dextrose in water (D_5W) and infused over 1 hour every 4 weeks. Dapsone may be given at a dose of 2 mg/kg/day (single dose) and comes in 25- and 100-mg tablets. Patients should commence this prophylaxis at the time of diagnosis and continue until 3 to 6 months after completion of therapy. Prophylaxis with TMP-SMX should be *discontinued 1 day prior to the administration of methotrexate* (due to interference with methotrexate excretion), and restarted after the serum methotrexate level has fallen to below 1×10^{-7} M. Temporary interruption of the doses may be necessary for prolonged marrow suppression or an increase in liver transaminases, rather than decreasing the dose of maintenance chemotherapy.

Prophylaxis for subacute bacterial endocarditis is recommended for patients with central venous catheters undergoing invasive procedures that could cause transient bacteremia and seeding of the catheter. Such procedures include dental cleaning or procedures, endotracheal intubation, and surgery involving the gastrointestinal or genitourinary tract. The standard regimen is the same as that recommended by the American Heart Association for children with congenital heart disease: amoxicillin 50 mg/kg (maximum 3 g) orally 1 hour prior to the procedure. Erythromycin or clindamycin may be given to penicillin-allergic patients (erythromycin ethylsuccinate 20 mg/kg PO, maximum 800 mg; or clindamycin 20 mg/kg PO or IV, maximum 600 mg) 1 to 2 hours prior to the procedure.

VIRAL PROPHYLAXIS

Common viral infections may be particularly virulent in immune-compromised children. These viruses include varicella zoster virus (VZV), herpes simplex virus (HSV), cytomegalovirus (CMV), Epstein-Barr virus (EBV), hepatitis types A and B virus, respiratory syncytial virus (RSV), and rubeola. Infection with these viruses may result in prolonged viral excretion, increased morbidity, or death. At the time of diagnosis, an immunization and infection history should be obtained. Obtain serologies for VZV, HSV, CMV, EBV, hepatitis (A, B, and C), and, in infants, RSV. These serologies should be checked yearly if negative at diagnosis.

The child exposed to **varicella zoster** who has a negative varicella immune status should receive varicella zoster immune globulin (VZIG) within 72 hours of exposure. The dosage is one vial (125 units) per 10 kg, to a maximum of five vials, intramuscularly. Administration of VZIG extends the incubation period from 21 to 28 days and decreases, but does not eliminate, the possibility of clinical infection with VZV. If VZIG is not available (from the American Red Cross), then intravenous immune globulin at 400 mg/kg can be given. Myelosuppressive chemotherapy may need to be stopped 7 days after the exposure and held until the end of the incubation period. The decision to hold chemotherapy during the incubation period should be based on the intensity of exposure, condition of the patient, and intensity of the chemotherapy. If varicella develops, stop chemotherapy and administer acyclovir (1500 mg/m^2/day divided q8h) for 5 to 10 days, until all lesions are crusted and no new lesions have appeared for 24 to 48 hours. Monitor renal and fluid status because of the nephrotoxicity of acyclovir. (Table 17–1 provides a formula for calculation of body surface area for drug dosing.)

Children with positive **herpes simplex virus** serology are at an increased risk of reactivation with subsequent courses of chemotherapy or

---

TABLE 17-1

CALCULATION OF BODY SURFACE AREA (BSA)*

$$\text{Formula: BSA (m}^2) = \frac{\sqrt{(ht[cm] + wt[kg])}}{60}$$

---

*Nomograms are also available to calculate BSA.

---

during and after a bone marrow transplant. Acyclovir administered pro-phylactically may prevent or decrease the severity of recurrent herpes infection and is generally recommended. A dose of 750 mg/m^2/day divided every 8 hours intravenously is recommended during periods of marked neutropenia. It can also be given orally, though the dose should be increased.

Prevention of **CMV** is critical in CMV-seronegative patients who are candidates for a bone marrow transplant. They should receive CMV-negative blood products or leukocyte-depleted blood products (per institutional practice). Certain patients may receive prophylaxis or treatment with ganciclovir in the peri-transplant period.

Immunizations
For general guidelines on passive immunization of the child with cancer, see Table 17-2.

TABLE 17-2

PASSIVE IMMUNIZATION OF THE CHILD WITH CANCER WHO IS ON CHEMOTHERAPY

Hepatitis A	Immune globulin 0.02 ml/kg IM, maximum dose of 2 ml. Given within 14 days of exposure. Good personal hygiene, hand washing.
Hepatitis B	**Previously unvaccinated children:** HBIG 0.06 ml/kg IM within 48 hours of exposure, maximum dose 5 ml. Start first of three-vaccine series. **Previously vaccinated children:** Known nonresponder (or unknown status), HBIG IM + vaccine. HBIG should be given within 24–48 hours and vaccine series initiated within 7 days.
Measles	Immune globulin 0.5 ml/kg IM, maximum dose 15 ml. Give within 6 days of exposure, regardless of previous immunization status.
Varicella	VZIG 1 vial/10 kg IM, maximum 5 vials. Given within 48 hours of exposure for maximum effect, up to 96 hours postexposure.
Tuberculosis	Isoniazid 10 mg/kg/day PO, maximum of 300 mg/day for 12 months. If patient is noncompliant, can change dose to twice weekly directly-observed therapy (20–30 mg/kg/day to maximum of 900 mg/day, preferably after 1 month of daily therapy).

Abbreviations: HBIG = hepatitis B immune globulin; VZIG = varicella zoster immune globulin.

TABLE 17–3

IMMUNIZATION OF THE CHILD WITH CANCER WHO IS ON THERAPY

DPT or DTaP	Recommended at appropriate age intervals in unimmunized children (routine boosters can be deferred)
Polio	OPV contraindicated; IPV is safe
MMR	Contraindicated
Pneumococcus, meningococcus	Recommended at appropriate age intervals, especially if asplenic
HIB	Recommended at appropriate age intervals in unimmunized children
HBV	Recommended at start of therapy if titer negative, if patient likely to receive blood products (recommended with HBIG for exposures)
Influenza	Recommended seasonally
Varicella	Recommended in ALL, maintenance (per the literature). Consider in other "lower risk" diagnoses. *Not FDA approved for use in children with cancer.*

Abbreviations: DPT = diphtheria–pertussis–tetanus; DTaP = diphtheria–tetanus–acellular pertussis; OPV = oral polio vaccine; IPV = inactivated polio virus; MMR = measles–mumps-rubella; HIB = *Haemophilus influenzae* type B vaccine; HBV = hepatitis B vaccine; HBIG = hepatitis B immune globulin; ALL = acute lymphoblastic leukemia; FDA = Food and Drug Administration.

Patients receiving chemotherapy, or who are otherwise immune compromised, should not receive live virus vaccines (measles–mumps–rubella and oral polio). Siblings or household contacts should not receive the oral polio vaccine. All other vaccines may continue as scheduled, though titers should be checked at completion of treatment because of the potential of loss of protective antibody titers as a result of immune suppressive therapy. Boosters or full reimmunization may be needed after completion of therapy, whether immunization occurred prior to or during therapy (see Table 17–3).

FUNGAL PROPHYLAXIS

Fungal prophylaxis is indicated in severely myelosuppressed patients. Mouth care is recommended routinely for the prevention and or treatment of mouth sores and yeast infection. Mycostatin oral swish and swallow (5 to 10 ml BID) or clotrimazole troches (1 BID, suck for 20 minutes) are routinely recommended. Fluconazole (3 to 6 mg/kg/day PO or IV) may be indicated in patients who are noncompliant with oral Mycostatin, unable to tolerate oral medications, or at very high risk of developing infection (acute myelogenous leukemia, high-risk acute lymphoblastic leukemia [ALL], ALL relapse, etc.). The most common fungal infections in patients receiving intensive chemotherapy include candidiasis and aspergillosis. Efforts to prevent invasive fungal disease (especially *Aspergillus* species, an airborne organism) include respiratory isolation, use of laminar airflow rooms, and use of high-efficiency particulate air (HEPA) filters. Patients should not have live plants in the room, play in dirt or gardens, or be in proximity to construction work. Several prophylactic regimens against invasive fungal disease in high-risk patients are being investigated and include administration of amphotericin B intravenously, fluconazole, or voriconazole during periods of severe, prolonged neutropenia.

ANTIEMETICS

Antiemetics are an important component of the supportive care regimen for patients receiving chemotherapy or radiation. Many of the common chemotherapeutic agents cause nausea and vomiting (Table 17–4). There are three types of antineoplastic drug–induced nausea and vomiting: anticipatory, acute, and delayed. Anticipatory emesis occurs before antineoplastic agents are administered and may be a result of nausea and vomiting experienced during previous cycles of antineoplastic therapy. Acute emesis occurs on day 1 of treatment and delayed emesis occurs on days 2 to 5 post-therapy. Poor control of nausea and vomiting may prolong or result in hospitalization or lead to dehydration or electrolyte abnormalities.

Serotonin (5-HT_3) receptor blocking agents are indicated for the prevention of nausea and vomiting associated with highly or moderate emetogenic chemotherapy. Cytotoxic chemotherapy appears to be associated with serotonin release from the enterochromaffin cells of the small intestine. The release of serotonin may stimulate the vagal afferents through the 5-HT_3 receptors and initiate vomiting. Serotonin antagonists block the 5-HT_3 receptors and inhibit vomiting. 5-HT_3 receptors are located both peripherally (vagal nerve terminals) and centrally in the chemoreceptor trigger zone. The drugs may have both peripheral and central effects.

DOSAGE AND ADMINISTRATION

The dosage and administration of serotonin antagonists is dependent on the emetogenicity of specific chemotherapeutic agents. Table 17–5 provides guidelines for the administration of ondansetron.

Continuous-infusion ondansetron can also be administered. The patient should receive 0.1 mg/kg (maximum 8 mg) prior to chemotherapy then 0.45 mg/kg/day (maximum 24 mg/day, 1 mg/hour) continuously until chemotherapy is completed.

If a patient continues to vomit after chemotherapy, ondansetron may be continued up to 24 hours after the chemotherapy has been discontinued. The goal of this therapy is to prevent inadequate caloric intake and/or dehydration. Ondansetron may be continued after administration of methotrexate until the serum level is cleared (1×10^{-7} M).

Ondansetron also comes in an oral form (4- and 8-mg tablets) and may be used at home for the prevention or treatment of nausea and vomiting with mildly emetogenic outpatient chemotherapy or radiation, or for delayed or prolonged emesis.

Granisetron is another serotonin antagonist used in the management of nausea and vomiting for children with cancer. The dose is 10 μg/kg IV 30

TABLE 17-4

QUICK GUIDE TO COMMON CHEMOTHERAPY DRUGS

DRUG CATEGORY	DRUG	TUMORS	ADVERSE AFFECTS	MONITORING
Alkylators	Carboplatin	Brain, sarcomas	Renal, hearing, N&V, BM	Cr, PO$_4$, lytes, (K, Ca, Mg), GFR, audio, I&O
	Cisplatin	NBL, osteo, germ cell, brain	N&V, BM (mild), renal, alopecia, neuro, hearing	Lytes, I&O
	Cyclophosphamide	ALL, lymphoma, NBL, sarcomas	BM, hemorrhagic cystitis, alopecia, N&V, SIADH	Lytes, I&O, ensure good UO, urine heme every void, (mesna, urine ketones)
	Ifosfamide	Sarcomas, germ cell, relapsed ALL	BM, N&V, cystitis, renal, alopecia, neuro	I&O, BUN, Cr, lytes, (Mg, Ca, PO$_4$), urine heme, GFR (mesna, urine ketones)
	Procarbazine	Hodgkin's, brain	MAO inhibitor, thrombocytopenia	Avoid certain foods (list available)
Antimetabolites	Cytarabine	AML, ALL, lymphoma	BM, N&V, GI, hepatic, fever, conjunctivitis	CBC, LFTs, Decadron eye drops with high dose
	Methotrexate	ALL, lymphoma, osteo	BM, mucositis, N&V, hepatic, renal, neuro	I&O, serum levels (plot), BUN, Cr, GFR (per protocol), mouth care, leucovorin rescue
	6-Thioguanine, 6-Mercaptopurine	ALL, AML	BM, hepatic	LFTs

	Drug	Indications	Side Effects	Monitoring
Antibiotics	Adriamycin/daunomycin	ALL, AML, lymphoma, osteo, most solid tumors, NBL	BM, mucositis, N&V, vesicant, cardiac	CBC, PE, echo
	Dactinomycin	Wilms', sarcomas	BM, mucositis, N&V, vesicant	LFTs, CBC
	Bleomycin	Hodgkin's, germ cell	Lung, skin, mucositis, vesicant	CXR, PFTs, pulse oximetry
Alkaloids	Vincristine	ALL, lymphoma, most solid tumors	Hepatic, vesicant constipation, peripheral neuropathy, SIADH, alopecia	LFTs, lytes, PE, CBC, stool softener, fluids
	Vinblastine	Hodgkin's, histiocytosis	Hepatic, BM, constipation, peripheral neuropathy	I&O, lytes, stool softener, fluids
	Etoposide	ALL, AML, lymphoma, NBL, brain, sarcomas	BM, N&V, BP, alopecia, mucositis, 2nd malignancy	I&O, slow IV infusion; monitor BP, CBC
Miscellaneous	Asparaginase	ALL, lymphoma	Hepatic, pancreatitis, diabetes, anaphylaxis	LFTs, coags, urine glucose, amylase, check site 1 hour post-IM
	Prednisone/Decadron	ALL, AML	HTN, diabetes, increased appetite, fluid retention, gastritis, mood lability	Urine glucose, BP, I&O, antacids/H2 blockers

Abbreviations: N&V = nausea & vomiting; BM = bone marrow suppression; Cr = creatinine; lytes = electrolytes; GFR = glomerular filtration rate; Audio = audiogram; I&O = intake and output; NBL = neuroblastoma; osteo = osteosarcoma; ALL = acute lymphoblastic leukemia; SIADH = syndrome of inappropriate secretion of antidiuretic hormone; UO = urinary output; BUN = blood urea nitrogen; MAO = monoamine oxidase; AML = acute myelogenous leukemia; GI = gastrointestinal; CBC = complete blood count; LFTs = liver function tests; PE = pulmonary edema; echo = echocardiography; CXR = chest x-ray; PFTs = pulmonary function tests; BP = blood pressure; coags = coagulation profiles; HTN = hypertension; H2 = histamine-2.

17

ANTIEMETICS

TABLE 17–5

ONDANSETRON DOSING GUIDELINES

EMETOGENIC POTENTIAL	CHEMOTHERAPY DRUG/DOSAGE	ONDANSETRON DOSE
High (>90%)	Cisplatin (>50 mg/m^2) Cytarabine (>1000 mg/m^2) Cyclophosphamide (>1500 mg/m^2)	0.45 mg/kg 30 min prechemotherapy, then q24h
Moderate-High (60–90%)	Cisplatin (<50 mg/m^2) Doxorubicin (Adriamycin) Cytarabine (250–1000 mg/m^2) Dactinomycin Methotrexate (>250 mg/m^2)	0.45 mg/kg 30 min prechemotherapy, then q24h
Moderate (30–60%)	Doxorubicin (<60 mg/m^2) Cyclophosphamide (<750 mg/m^2) Idarubicin Carboplatin Ifosfamide	0.15 mg/kg 30 min prechemotherapy, then q8h × 3 doses
Moderate-Low (10–30%)	Cytarabine (<250 mg/m^2) Etoposide Hydroxyurea 6-MP Methotrexate (50–250 mg/m^2) Thiotepa Vinblastine Radiation therapy (daily)	0.15 mg/kg 30 min prechemotherapy
Low (<10%)	Bleomycin 6-TG (50–250 mg/m^2) Vincristine Methotrexate (<50 mg/m^2) Fludarabine	Consider; no antiemetic or promethazine *or* metoclopromide + diphenhydramine

minutes prior to administration of chemotherapy. Its safety and efficacy . profile is similar to that of ondansetron.

SIDE EFFECTS OF SEROTONIN ANTAGONISTS

- Common adverse effects: diarrhea, headache, constipation, hepatic effects (mild transaminase elevations), rash, sedation
- Serious adverse effects: irritable bowel syndrome, ileus, vascular occlusive events, syncope, seizures

ADJUNCTIVE THERAPY

Adjunctive therapy for persistent nausea and vomiting includes the following:

1. Dexamethasone (0.1 mg/kg/dose or 5 to 10 mg/m^2) may be added to increase the antiemetic potency of ondansetron. Do not use in patients receiving steroids as chemotherapy.

2. Diphenhydramine and metoclopramide (1 mg/kg/dose PO/IV of each, maximum 50 mg/dose) may be administered every 4 hours if needed.

3. Promethazine (0.25 to 0.5 mg/kg/dose) may also be added to the above. (**Caution:** Extrapyramidal symptoms [EPS] occur with high doses; administer with diphenhydramine to prevent EPS.)

4. Lorazepam 0.1 mg/kg/dose PO/IV (maximum single dose 2 mg) may be added for anticipatory nausea and vomiting or as adjunctive therapy.

5. Cannabinoids have been used in adults to treat nausea related to chemotherapy. No data are available for use in children. but they have been used successfully in adolescents. Dose is 5 mg/m^2 1 to 3 hours prior to chemotherapy, then 5 mg/m^2 q2–4h (can be increased to effective dose, maximum 15 mg/m^2/dose). Smoking cannabinoids should be discouraged because of possible impurities or exposure to fungal organisms.

GUIDELINES FOR USE OF HEMATOPOIETIC GROWTH FACTORS IN CHILDREN WITH CANCER

Several hematopoietic growth factors have been approved for clinical use and include granulocyte colony-stimulating factor (G-CSF; filgrastim) granulocyte-macrophage colony-stimulating factor (GM-CSF; sargramostim), and erythropoietin (EPO; epoetin alfa). The indications and doses for each of these growth factors may depend on the intensity of the chemotherapy regimen and the current data on its use in children. When no specific recommendations for use of these factors are made in a study or protocol, the following guidelines may prove useful.

G-CSF (FILGRASTIM)
Indications
G-CSF stimulates the proliferation, maturation, and function of granulocytes. Although the absolute neutrophil count (ANC) may fall with G-CSF as without it, the duration of neutropenia is typically shorter.

Primary Administration

1. G-CSF should be given to patients receiving multiagent chemotherapy who are expected to experience a high incidence of febrile neutropenia or severe, prolonged neutropenia (ANC <500/μl for 7 or more days).

2. G-CSF should not be given on the same days on which patients are given myelosuppressive chemotherapy and/or radiation therapy.

3. G-CSF administration may be warranted in patients at high risk for infectious complications as a result of pre-existing neutropenia, extensive prior chemotherapy, prior irradiation to areas containing large amounts of bone marrow, history of febrile neutropenia while receiving earlier chemotherapy, or conditions increasing the risk of infection

17

USE OF HEMATOPOIETIC GROWTH FACTORS IN CHILDREN WITH CANCER

(e.g., open wounds, active infections), or when the clinical situation is deemed appropriate.

Secondary Administration

1. Secondary administration of G-CSF is reserved for patients after a documented incident of febrile neutropenia in an earlier chemotherapy cycle. The goal is to decrease the occurrence of febrile neutropenia in subsequent chemotherapy cycles.
2. G-CSF may also be considered if the patient's course of neutropenia has been prolonged, causing dose reduction or delay of chemotherapy.
3. G-CSF can be used to treat fever and neutropenia (ANC <500/μl) as an adjunct to antibiotics in ill patients experiencing pneumonia, hypotension, multiorgan dysfunction (sepsis), or fungal infection.

Dose and Route of Administration

1. The recommended dose is 5 μg/kg/day SQ. There are no data to support higher dosing. If the patient warrants IV G-CSF, the dose may need to be increased.
2. *Subcutaneous* administration is the preferred route of administration for G-CSF.
3. If the patient is severely thrombocytopenic and subcutaneous injections are causing swelling and/or bruising, G-CSF may be given IV over 30 to 60 minutes at a concentration greater than or equal to 15 μg/ml. G-CSF must be diluted or mixed in D_5W ONLY. The use of any other diluent may cause G-CSF precipitation or pharmacologic inactivation.

Duration

1. G-CSF should be started between 24 and 72 hours after the last dose of myelosuppressive chemotherapy or radiation.
2. G-CSF should be continued until the ANC is greater than 5000/μl for 1 to 2 days, AFTER the expected neutrophil nadir from the chemotherapy. Specific protocols may call for a different ANC.

Monitoring

Once G-CSF is initiated, a complete blood count (CBC) and differential should be monitored at least twice a week.

Adverse Effects

The most common side effects of G-CSF are bone pain and elevation of uric acid, lactate dehydrogenase (LDH), and alkaline phosphatase. Occasionally, G-CSF has been reported to cause fever, nausea and vomiting, diarrhea, splenomegaly, and erythema at the injection site.

GM-CSF (SARGRAMOSTIM)
Indications
GM-CSF stimulates the proliferation and maturation of granulocytes and macrophages. It has an important role in post–bone marrow transplant recovery.

Primary Administration
1. GM-CSF is recommended in patients who have just received an autologous or allogeneic bone marrow transplant.
2. GM-CSF is recommended following peripheral blood stem cell transplantation.

Secondary Administration
1. GM-CSF has been used following myelosuppressive chemotherapy that is expected to result in an ANC less than $500/\mu l$ for 7 or more days.
2. GM-CSF has also been used with myelodysplastic syndrome.

Dose and Route of Administration
The recommended dose is $250\ \mu g/m^2/day$ IV over 2 to 4 hours for both the prevention and treatment of engraftment delay. GM-CSF may also be given SQ.

Duration
1. When given after a bone marrow transplant, the first dose should be given within 2 to 4 hours, then doses given daily for 21 days or until the ANC is greater than $10,000/\mu l$.
2. GM-CSF should not be given within 24 hours of the last round of chemotherapy or within 12 hours of the last dose of radiation therapy.

Monitoring
A CBC with differential should be monitored at least twice a week. Monitor renal and hepatic function twice a week, or more often as clinically indicated. Because of possible fluid retention syndrome, monitor patients for weight gain, unbalanced intake and output, respiratory distress, and pleural or pericardial effusions.

Adverse Effects
Occasionally, GM-CSF may cause bone pain, leukocytosis, diarrhea, rash, headache, fever, arthralgias, chest pain, dyspnea, thrombocytopenia, and thrombophlebitis. Rarely, its use has been associated with fluid retention (peripheral edema, pleural or pericardial effusion, respiratory distress, renal failure), supraventricular arrhythmias, bundle-branch block, thrombosis, hypotension, facial flushing, and elevation of LDH, alkaline phosphatase, and/or transaminases.

RECOMBINANT HUMAN ERYTHROPOIETIN

Clinical trials are currently in progress to evaluate the safety and efficacy of EPO in chemotherapy-induced anemia in children. Adult trials are promising, particularly for patients receiving cisplatin-based regimens.

Indications

There are no proven indications for EPO in pediatric oncology. When its use is being considered, other causes of anemia (nutritional anemias, hemolysis, blood loss) should be assessed. Consideration for its use should be given in the following situations:

1. Refusal of blood transfusion based on religious beliefs
2. Anemia associated with radiation therapy
3. Anemia of chronic disease or secondary to very myelosuppressive chemotherapy

Dose and Route of Administration

1. The starting dose of EPO is 150 U/kg/dose SQ or IV three times a week. If there is no response within 2 to 4 weeks, the dose may be increased to 300 U/kg/dose. Titration to a lower dose may be indicated for an excessively elevated hemoglobin.
2. Adequate iron stores or supplementation may be necessary to ensure optimal response.

Duration

Continue EPO until the patient is considered to not be transfusion dependent. EPO may be given concurrently with chemotherapy or radiation.

Monitoring

Monitor CBC and reticulocyte count prior to initiation of EPO and weekly thereafter. Assess blood urea nitrogen, creatinine, and potassium every 2 to 4 weeks; ferritin every month; and blood pressure at every visit (at least every 2 to 4 weeks). EPO levels may be obtained prior to the start of therapy and may be useful in predicting response.

Adverse Effects

The most common side effects of EPO are hypertension, local pain at the injection site for SQ administration, headache, fever, and diarrhea. Occasionally, EPO has been associated with nausea, thrombosis of vascular access devices, flulike symptoms, and seizures.

SUGGESTED READING

Altman AJ, Wolff LJ. The prevention of infection. In: Ablin AR (ed), Supportive Care of Children with Cancer, 2nd ed. Baltimore: The Johns Hopkins University Press, 1997, pp 1–12.

Hastings C, Goes C, Wolff LJ. Immunization of the child with cancer. In: Ablin AR (ed), Supportive Care of Children with Cancer, 2nd ed. Baltimore: The Johns Hopkins University Press, 1997, pp 13–22.

Miller LL, Smith MA, Nagler CH. The role of hematopoietic cytokines in supportive care. In: Pizzo PA, Polpcak DG (eds), Principles and Practice of Pediatric Oncology, 3rd ed. Philadelphia: Lippincott–Raven, 1997, pp 1115–1165.

Sallan SE, Billet AL. Management of nausea and vomiting. In: Pizzo PA, Poplack DG (eds), Principles and Practice of Pediatric Oncology, 3rd ed. Philadelphia: Lippincott–Raven, 1997, pp 1201–1208.

CENTRAL VENOUS CATHETERS

Indwelling central venous catheters (CVCs) have been in use for the past 20 years and have revolutionized the care of children with cancer. Peripheral venous access can become increasingly difficult in young children, particularly if they are receiving chemotherapeutic agents that produce venous sclerosis. During the course of intensive therapy, children can also expect to need venous access for antibiotics, blood products, hydration, parenteral nutrition, pain medication, anesthesia, and supportive medications, including antiemetics.

18

Two major types of indwelling CVCs are used for children. Right atrial catheters are inserted via the subclavian, internal, or external jugular vein with a subcutaneous tunnel to an exit site on the anterior or lateral chest. These catheters typically are single or double lumen, and occasionally triple lumen. The most frequently used are Broviac and Hickman catheters. Totally implantable catheters, or "ports," are right atrial catheters that lead to reservoirs under the skin and are without external lumens. Older children and adolescents frequently prefer these ports because they are cosmetically more satisfactory, do not require routine care, and allow for easy bathing and swimming.

MAINTENANCE

Externalized catheters require daily heparin flushes, in addition to dressing changes three times a week. Sterile technique should always be used for accessing the CVC for blood draws or flushes and for external care. Mediports require less care, with heparin flushes at least monthly. No dressing changes are needed for implantable devices. Each institution should develop consistent sterile guidelines for the care of CVCs, to be followed by all the staff, the family members, and home health care agencies.

COMPLICATIONS

The major complications of CVCs are **infection** and **thrombosis**. A thrombus may also serve as a nidus of infection. An immune suppressed child with a CVC and fever should be presumed to be bacteremic (see Chapter 19, Central venous catheter infections). The most common organisms are coagulase-negative staphylococci. Empiric antibiotics should be administered after drawing cultures from each lumen of the CVC. Antibiotic therapy is usually successful in treating bacteremia associated with a CVC, infrequently necessitating removal of the line. Persistent bacteremia despite appropriate antibiotic coverage (48 hours) or signs of sepsis (hypotension, chills, persistent fever) warrant removal of the CVC.

If there is a site infection, the drainage should be cultured, and parenteral antibiotics administered with good local care of the exit site. Tunnel infections (tenderness, erythema, swelling along the internal tract) may require removal of the catheter if parenteral antibiotics do not result in resolution of the signs and symptoms. When evaluating a child with fever and a CVC, palpate along the tunnel to assess for tenderness or express drainage if infection is suspected. Site or tunnel infections with certain organisms (fungus, gram-negative organisms) may require surgical débridement with removal of the line. Fungemia from the line is always an indication for immediate line removal.

ASSESSMENT AND MANAGEMENT OF SEPSIS

A child who presents with or develops signs or symptoms of sepsis (fever, chills, rigors, hypotension) following access and flush of a CVC should be presumed to be bacteremic and possibly have a nidus of bacteria in the CVC. Cardiovascular compromise or collapse has been reported to occur in this setting. Following are guidelines for the assessment and management of the child with chills or fever following flush of the CVC.

1. Obtain peripheral intravenous access and do not use the CVC to administer fluids or medications or draw specimens for laboratory studies.
2. Blood cultures should be obtained from the CVC if possible, without flushing the line (which may ultimately clot). Blood cultures should be obtained peripherally if not obtainable centrally.
3. Administer a fluid bolus of 20 ml/kg of normal saline or lactated Ringer's solution over 30 to 60 minutes.
4. Start empiric broad-spectrum antibiotics (see guidelines Chapter 19).
5. Monitor vital signs carefully, including blood pressure.
6. Repeat fluid bolus as clinically indicated.
7. If the symptoms abate and the blood culture is negative at 24 hours, administer fluid bolus and attempt to withdraw blood and flush the line. If the line works well and there are no further signs or symptoms of sepsis, continue to use the CVC. Complete a full course of antibiotics.
8. If evidence of sepsis continues or blood cultures are positive, removal of the CVC may be necessary. Complete a full course of antibiotics. Consider not replacing the CVC at all, or at least until completion of antibiotics and recovery of the ANC.

ASSESSMENT AND MANAGEMENT OF THROMBOSIS

If a line does not flush easily or will not withdraw blood, the line may be clotted or be up against a vessel wall. Below are guidelines for assessment and treatment of a suspected CVC-associated thrombus.

1. Examine the catheter for any kinks in the tubing.
2. Reposition the child, flush the CVC with normal saline, and again attempt to withdraw blood. Have the child hold the hands above the head, turn, cough, or hold breath.

3. Obtain a radiographic study, such as a dye study, to evaluate for thrombus formation. Assess for sleeve thrombus, mechanical failure of the CVC, or migration of the catheter outside of the vessel.
4. If a thrombus is identified, administer a thrombolytic agent, such as tissue plasminogen activator t-PA (Alteplase) or urokinase, via the catheter. Instill one dose into each lumen, allow to dwell for 30 minutes. **Dosage** is as follows:
   a. **t-PA:** children less than 3 months, 0.25 mg/0.5 ml; children 3 months or older, 0.5 mg/1 ml per lumen
   b. **Urokinase** 5000 U/ml per lumen.
5. Attach an empty 3-ml syringe and attempt to withdraw blood. If successful, obtain blood work and flush line per protocol. If unsuccessful, instill a second dose of the thrombolytic agent and allow to dwell for 30 minutes. If this second dose fails, a 6- to 12-hour infusion should be considered. **Infusion dosage** is as follows:
   a. **t-PA:** 0.01 mg/kg/hour for 6 hours; if no clinical improvement, increase dose to 0.02 mg/kg/hour for 6 hours. A third infusion at 0.03 mg/kg/hour for 6 hours may be given.
   b. **Urokinase:** 200 units/kg/hour/lumen for 12 to 28 hours.
6. Obtain a repeat radiographic study to assess for improvement after instillation or infusion of thrombolytic agents.
7. Monitor the child for signs of sepsis because bacteria can be released into the bloodstream as the thrombus dissolves.
8. Remove the catheter if the thrombus is not able to be cleared after 24 to 48 hours.

18

COMPLICATIONS

SUGGESTED READING

Dillon PW, Weiner ES. Venous access devices in children. In: Ablin AR (ed), Supportive Care of Children with Cancer, 3rd ed. Baltimore: The Johns Hopkins University Press, 1997, pp 217–227.

MANAGEMENT OF FEVER IN THE CHILD WITH CANCER

FEVER AND NEUTROPENIA

Children with cancer are at an increased risk for serious bacterial, viral, and fungal infections. The single most important factor determining susceptibility is the number of circulating neutrophils. The risk of infection is directly related to the length and severity of neutropenia.

The absolute neutrophil count (ANC) is calculated by multiplying the percentage of neutrophils (segmented neutrophils + bands) by the total white blood cell (WBC) count. For example:

$$\text{WBC} = 1000/\mu l, \text{ segs} = 10, \text{ bands} = 10$$
$$20\% \ (0.2) \times 1000 = 200/\mu l$$

The severity of neutropenia is determined by the ANC:

ANC less than $1000/\mu l$ is defined as mild neutropenia
ANC less than $500/\mu l$ represents moderate neutropenia
ANC less than $200/\mu l$ represents severe neutropenia

Fever is defined as a single temperature of 38.5°C or two temperatures of 38.0°C or higher within a 1- to 2-hour period, taken per axilla, orally, or by tympanic probe. Rectal temperatures should never be taken in potentially neutropenic children.

Every oncology patient who presents with fever and neutropenia is considered septic until proven otherwise. These children may have fever as their only symptom of infection. A careful clinical examination is critical because their status may change quickly and dramatically.

Septic shock is caused by overwhelming infection from microorganisms in the blood that results in circulatory failure, inadequate tissue perfusion, and hypotension. Symptoms of septic shock are hypotension, tachycardia, tachypnea, clammy extremities, decreased urine output, and deterioration of mental status.

The most common organisms causing sepsis are

- Gram-positive: coagulase-negative and coagulase-positive *Staphylococcus*, *Streptococcus viridans*
- Gram-negative: *Escherichia coli*, *Enterobacter* species, *Klebsiella* species, *Pseudomonas* species, *Serratia* species, *Acinetobacter* species

INITIAL EVALUATION (FIG. 19–1)

1. **History and physical examination**: includes determination of vital signs and evaluation for shock. Conduct a meticulous physical examination with particular attention to sites of occult infection: oral cavity and skin, including perianal area. Even subtle evidence of inflam-

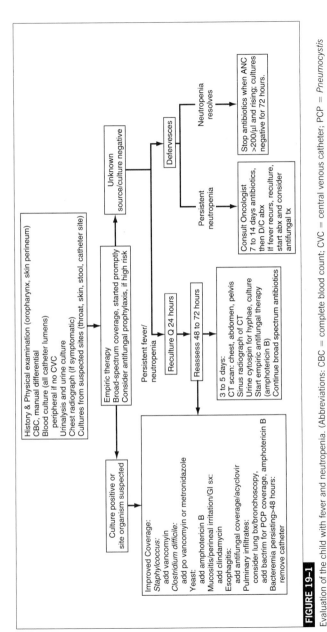

FIGURE 19-1

Evaluation of the child with fever and neutropenia. (Abbreviations: CBC = complete blood count; CVC = central venous catheter; PCP = *Pneumocystis carinii* pneumonia; CT = computed tomography; ANC = absolute neutrophil count.)

mation may provide a possible source of infection (faint redness, tenderness, or minimal discharge).

2. The **laboratory evaluation** includes a complete blood count with manual differential to determine the ANC. Samples for blood cultures are taken from each lumen of a central venous catheter (CVC); a peripheral culture sample is necessary if the child does not have a central line or a sample is not obtainable from the central line. Remember not to flush the CVC if the patient is febrile, chilled, or hypotensive following access (see Chapter 18).
3. Urinalysis and urine culture should be done.
4. A chest radiograph should be taken if any pulmonary signs or symptoms are present.
5. Culture and stain samples should be taken from suspicious skin sites of infection: oropharynx, skin, and catheter sites. If diarrhea is present, then culture stool and send a sample for *Clostridium difficile* toxin.
6. The child with tenderness over the sinuses should have a diagnostic imaging study to evaluate for sinusitis (plain radiographs or computed tomography [CT]).
7. Lumbar punctures are not routinely done as part of an initial septic work-up. **If a lumbar puncture seems indicated initially, contact the pediatric hematologist/oncologist immediately for assessment. Evaluation for increased cerebral pressure may be necessary by imaging in some patients prior to lumbar puncture.**

INITIAL MANAGEMENT OF THE FEBRILE NEUTROPENIC CHILD

Broad-spectrum antibiotics must be started immediately. All organisms are potentially pathogenic. Antibiotics should be chosen based on microbial prevalence and antibiotic sensitivity patterns at each institution. Many combinations of antimicrobials are effective; however, drug resistance may develop in some centers.

Various antibiotic combinations that are used for fever and neutropenia in immune-compromised hosts are as follows:

1. Aminoglycoside plus an antipseudomonal β-lactam drug: ceftazidime 100 mg/kg/day IV divided q8h + tobramycin 7.5 mg/kg/day IV divided q8h
2. Extended-spectrum penicillin plus antipseudomonal aminoglycoside: azlocillin, mezlocillin, piperacillin, or ticarcillin + tobramycin
3. Monotherapy with a third-generation cephalosporin or imipenem (depending on institutional pathogens and susceptibilities):
   a. Cefoperazone 100 mg/kg/day IV divided q8h *or*
   b. Ceftazidime 100 mg/kg/day IV divided q8h *or*
   c. Imipenem 50 mg/kg/day IV divided q6–8h *or*
   d. Cefepime 150 mg/kg/day IV divided q8h

19

FEVER AND NEUTROPENIA

Aminoglycoside levels should be monitored, especially because the patient is likely to be receiving other nephrotoxic drugs. Monitor electrolytes, fluid balance, and renal function studies, and ensure adequate hydration.

MODIFICATION OF INITIAL TREATMENT

This broad-spectrum approach may be altered, or added to, if a source of infection is found to explain the initial fever, or the fever persists for more than 1 week. If the source of the infection is a catheter site, then vancomycin may be added. If the source is perianal, gingival, or intra-abdominal, then anaerobic coverage is added (clindamycin, metronidazole).

Vancomycin is the most effective antibiotic against increasingly frequent plasmid-mediated, β-lactam–resistant (methicillin-resistant *Staphylococcus aureus*) gram-positive bacteria and against all coagulase-negative staphylococci. No excess morbidity arises from a delay in adding it after the microbiology or clinical course warrants it. Vancomycin should *not* be part of empiric antibiotics unless the institutional experience and susceptibility patterns require it. However, it should be part of the initial therapy in a child with AML and fever due to the increased likelihood of *Streptococcus viridans* infection.

Protracted fever carries the risk of a second infection. Antibiotic-induced colitis may occur after any antibiotic. *Clostridium difficile* overgrowth runs the spectrum from asymptomatic to mild diarrhea to abdominal pain to pseudomembranous colitis with peritoneal signs and mucosal erosions. Because *C. difficile* is a normal bowel inhabitant, the toxin must be documented to diagnose this condition. Treatment is either oral vancomycin 125 mg QID or metronidazole 250 mg QID. Abdominal pain may also be from aerobic gram-negative bacteria, *Enterococcus* (which no cephalosporin covers in vivo), and anaerobes.

CENTRAL VENOUS CATHETER INFECTIONS

Coagulase-negative (non–*S. aureus*) staphylococci are the usual infective agent. However, resistant *Corynebacterium, Bacillus* species, atypical mycobacteria, fungi, and even gram-negative bacteria, especially *Acinetobacter* and *Pseudomonas*, can infect the neutropenic child.

Management

Most catheter-related bacteremias clear with appropriate antibiotics and do not require catheter removal.

1. In multilumen devices, the antibiotic infusion should be rotated among the ports because infection may not be limited to one lumen.
2. Daily blood culture samples should be taken while the child is febrile or if growth is present (from each lumen of CVC).
3. If bacteremia persists for more than 48 hours of appropriate therapy, then the catheter should be removed. If *Candida albicans* or *Bacillus* species are isolated, then the catheter should be removed promptly

because these organisms frequently fail any antibiotic or antifungal treatment.

4. Catheter site infections can be difficult to eradicate, especially when gram-negative bacteria, mycobacteria, or fungi are present. Frequently, the catheter must come out. Vancomycin may be added empirically for an infected site, assuming a possible staph infection.

5. If another implantable device, such as an Ommaya reservoir, is present, it may be necessary to tap it to determine if it may be the source of infection (only *after* consultation with the pediatric hematologist/oncologist). A lumbar puncture is also a consideration if a ventriculo-peritoneal shunt or Ommaya reservoir is present. **A CT scan may be important to obtain, depending on the clinical presentation, such as signs of shunt failure (headache, neurologic changes).**

6. Once the neutropenic child is afebrile for 24 hours, cultures are negative, and there is evidence of bone marrow recovery (increase in ANC for 2 or more consecutive days, level at least to 200/μl and rising), the antibiotics can be discontinued.

TREATMENT OF INFECTION
Positive Bacterial Blood Culture

The most common bacterial pathogens in neutropenic hosts are coagulase-negative and coagulase-positive *Staphylococcus* species and *Streptococcus* species, including *S. viridans*. When a pathogen has been identified, ensure appropriate antibiotic coverage by susceptibility patterns, and continue broad-spectrum coverage until the patient is afebrile and has evidence of bone marrow recovery. When the child is afebrile and the ANC recovers, antibiotics can be tailored to the specific agent for a full 10- to 14-day course.

Viral Infection

For documented infection with herpes simplex virus, treat with acyclovir 750 mg/m^2/day IV divided q8h. Infection with varicella zoster virus is potentially life threatening and should be treated with higher doses of acyclovir, 1500 mg/m^2/day IV divided q8h. Ensure adequate hydration and urine flow. Oral acyclovir should not be given because its bioavailability is unpredictable. If cytomegalovirus (CMV) is documented, initiate treatment with ganciclovir 10 mg/kg/day IV divided q12h in addition to CMV immune globulin.

Pneumocystis carinii Infection

For documented or highly suspected infection with *Pneumocystis carinii*, treat with trimethoprim–sulfamethoxazole (TMP-SMX): TMP 15 to 20 mg/kg/day and SMX 75 to 100 mg/kg/day PO or IV divided q8–12h for at least 14 days. If this therapy is not tolerated, treat with pentamidine 4 mg/kg/day IV or TMP 20 mg/kg/day divided q6h plus dapsone 100 mg/day PO for 21 days.

NEW SITE INFECTIONS

Persistent fever and neutropenia may be associated with the development of new sites of infection as a result of continued severe immune suppression. Particular symptoms may provide clues to site and potential pathogen.

Burning retrosternal pain may be esophagitis from *Candida* species or herpes simplex virus. Cytotoxic treatment may also cause severe pain as a result of mucosal erosions. Empiric amphotericin B or acyclovir, or both, may be needed. Esophagitis may also be bacterial, often resulting from gram-positive aerobes.

Pulmonary infiltrates may be from resistant bacteria, *P. carinii*, fungi, or viruses. Neutropenic patients whose ANCs are rising may develop new infiltrates that simply represent inflammation at previously unrecognized infection sites. If the ANC has not increased and the neutropenia has lasted less than a week, then bacteria are the most likely culprit, and antibiotic management may need to be augmented. If the neutropenia persists for more than a week, and/or the patient is at particularly high risk because of the underlying disease and degree of immune suppression, then fungal species are likely. Start therapeutic doses of amphotericin B with the diagnostic evaluation. Common occult foci include sinuses (diagnose with CT), kidneys, (ultrasound, CT, urine hyphae), lungs (CT), liver (CT), and skin. The risks and benefits of open lung biopsy and pursuing an aggressive diagnostic evaluation must be judged. It is important to remember that the child is likely to become very ill rapidly, and this decision must be made expeditiously by the pediatric oncologist, surgeon, radiologist, and pulmonologist. Bronchoalveolar lavage or induced sputum may find *P. carinii*, viruses, or fungi. Intravenous TMP–SMX should be initiated for presumed *P. carinii*.

TREATMENT OF PERSISTENT FEVER AND NEUTROPENIA

When fever and neutropenia persist for 3 or more days, a new assessment should be made to determine if a new bacterial, fungal, viral, or parasitic infection has developed. A meticulous physical examination, repeat laboratory assessment, and radiographic studies assessing for deep-seated infections are done at this time. For patients at particularly high risk for invasive fungal infection (acute myelogenous leukemia [AML], relapsed acute lymphoblastic leukemia, bone marrow transplant recipient), this evaluation should start at 72 hours of persistent fever and neutropenia. In patients with other levels of risk, the evaluation typically begins after 5 days of persistent fever and neutropenia. Fungal culture samples should be sent from the blood, urine (including cytology for staining), stool, and any suspicious skin site. Radiographic studies need to include CT of the sinuses, chest, abdomen, and pelvis to search for evidence of occult infection.

Empiric antifungal therapy prevents fungal overgrowth in patients with prolonged neutropenia. It also provides early treatment of clinically occult infections. Recent clinical trials have found that antifungal treatment of children with persistent or recurrent fever reduced morbidity and mortality from invasive fungal disease. This is especially true in patients with profound neutropenia not receiving antifungal prophylaxis. Amphotericin B at 0.6 mg/kg/day is used empirically. The dose may be increased to 1 mg/kg/day in the child in whom fungus is documented (positive blood culture, biopsy, or hyphae on stains) or highly suspected (pulmonary infiltrate, lesions in the liver and/or spleen, skin nodules, or sinus disease, especially with erosive bone changes).

Although amphotericin B is the most active antifungal agent, it has severe toxicity. Nephrotoxicity is the most frequent and severe problem. Fever, chills, nausea, thrombocytopenia, metabolic abnormalities, hypokalemia, electrolyte disturbances, and hepatic toxicity can also occur. To treat, and possibly prevent, some of these complications, several measures are taken. Patients with renal toxicity may benefit by receiving pre- and post-infusion normal saline boluses and/or diuretics. Premedications such as acetaminophen, diphenhydramine, and meperidine may be given to treat or prevent acute symptoms related to the infusion (fever, chills, rigors, nausea). Hydrocortisone can also be added to amphotericin to address infusion-related toxicity. Lipid formulations of amphotericin B may be indicated for severe renal or infusion-related toxicity, or failure to respond. The duration of antibiotic and antifungal treatment depends on the clinical response. Some authorities continue until the neutropenia resolves, and others treat for a full course (at least 14 days). Therapy may be needed until the child has completed all immune suppressive treatment. If the fever persists, then a search for other viral or bacterial superinfections must ensue. Recurrent malignant disease should also be considered.

Granulocyte colony-stimulating factor may be indicated in fever and neutropenia, especially in the setting of sepsis or suspected invasive fungal disease.

FEVER IN THE NON-NEUTROPENIC ONCOLOGY PATIENT

Follow all the same measures for a careful examination and laboratory studies as in the febrile neutropenic patient. If the child has a CVC, begin antibiotic therapy with a third-generation cephalosporin (e.g., ceftazidime 100 mg/kg/day divided q8h). Some patients may be given antibiotics and monitored as outpatients, seen daily until afebrile and blood cultures are negative for 72 hours. The patient should also be assessed for a dropping WBC/ANC if persistently febrile or if cultures are positive, in which case hospital admission may be warranted. Some patients with fever and moderate neutropenia (ANC ≥200/μl with anticipated short recovery) without high-risk factors (no concerning physical findings, normal blood pressure, remission status, diagnosis not AML or post–bone marrow transplantation) may be treated with similar guidelines.

Patients without central venous lines may be watched carefully and cultures obtained, without antibiotics being administered. Again, close and frequent observation is crucial, as is the involvement of the pediatric oncologist. The entire picture, consisting of the history, physical, underlying diagnosis, status of disease and therapy, laboratory studies, and patient compliance, needs to be taken into account when making the therapeutic plan.

PREVENTION OF INFECTION

Hand washing is the most important method of prevention of infection. Reverse isolation does not prevent infection after the onset of neutropenia. Most infections arise from the patient's endogenous biologic flora. Wearing masks and gloves does nothing to protect the child from such infections; however, they may reduce exposure to nosocomial infections. Children with very severe (ANC $<100/\mu l$) and/or prolonged (≥ 7 days) neutropenia should stay in high-efficiency particulate air (HEPA)-filtered rooms while hospitalized to decrease their exposure to nosocomial or community infections.

Prophylactic antibiotics may help. TMP-SMX can decrease the incidence of *P. carinii* infections. Mouth care with antibacterial and antifungal agents also reduces the incidence of oral infections. Acyclovir prophylaxis decreases the severity of herpes simplex infections.

SUGGESTED READING

Freifeld AG, Walsh TJ, Pizzo PA. Infectious complications in the pediatric cancer patient. In: Pizzo PA, Polack DG (eds), Principles and Practice of Pediatric Oncology, 3rd ed. Philadelphia: Lippincott–Raven, 1997, pp 1069–1114.

Wolff LJ, Ablin AR, Altman AJ, Johnson FL. The management of fever. In: Ablin AR (ed), Supportive Care of Children with Cancer, 2nd ed. Baltimore: The Johns Hopkins University Press, 1997, pp 23–36.

ONCOLOGIC EMERGENCIES

SUPERIOR VENA CAVA SYNDROME

Superior vena cava syndrome (SVCS) refers to compression and obstruction of flow of the vena cava and may include tracheal compression (more commonly seen in pediatrics). Superior vena cava syndrome (SVCS) is seen in 12% of pediatric patients on presentation with anterior mediastinal masses. Malignant tumors are the most common primary cause of SVCS; most are non-Hodgkin's lymphoma. Other causes include mediastinal granulomas (histoplasmosis), aortic aneurysms, vascular thrombosis complicating cardiovascular surgery for coronary heart disease, shunting for hydrocephalus, catheterizations, and infections (tuberculosis, syphilis).

The superior vena cava (SVC) is a thin-walled vessel with low intraluminal pressure, prone to thrombosis, surrounded by the thymus and nodes that drain the right side and lower left side of the chest. Part of the SVC also is in the pericardial reflection. Lymph nodes or thymus may become enlarged from infection or tumor involvement and compress the SVC. Adjacent pericardium and coronary and collateral vessels can become clotted. Compression, clotting, and edema lead to diminished airflow and blood flow (trachea and right mainstem bronchus are less rigid in children).

EVALUATION

Symptoms of SVCS include cough, hoarseness, dyspnea, orthopnea, chest pain, anxiety, confusion, lethargy, headache, visual changes, syncope, and fullness in the ears. Symptoms may be aggravated by the supine position.

Signs include swelling; plethora; cyanosis of face, neck, and upper extremities; diaphoresis; wheezing; stridor; engorged chest wall vessels; brachial veins remaining full with raising of the right arm; and pleural and/or pericardial effusions. Signs/symptoms may progress rapidly over several days.

A chest radiograph usually shows a mass in the anterior mediastinum, tracheal compression, and possibly effusions. The history, physical examination, and chest radiograph often are enough for differential diagnosis and determination of a plan. Histoplasmosis can usually be ruled out as a possibility in nonendemic areas (>1:32 antibody titer suggests infection). Vascular problems can usually be determined on radiographic imaging. Malignancies to be considered include lymphoma, leukemia, dysgerminoma, and seminoma (may see elevated α-fetoprotein, human chorionic gonadotropin).

DIAGNOSIS

Diagnostic procedures in general are poorly tolerated. General anesthesia may cause cardiovascular and/or respiratory compromise by increasing abdominal tone and decreasing respiratory muscle tone and lung volume. Sedatives can also decrease venous return and should be used cautiously.

The least invasive means of diagnostic testing should be done. Studies to be obtained may include peripheral blood counts/review of smear, bone marrow aspirate and/or biopsy, lymph node aspiration, chest computed tomography (CT) (tracheal size), and echocardiogram.

THERAPY

Children should be under close observation in the intensive care unit, with elevation of the head, continuous cardiovascular and respiratory monitoring, and pulse oximetry. Avoid sedation.

Because of the life-threatening nature of the situation, it may be necessary to initiate empiric therapy for suspected malignancy. Chemotherapy may be started with prednisone 40 to 60 mg/m^2/day divided QID. Steroids, cyclophosphamide, vincristine, or anthracyclines have been given in this situation to children with suspected leukemia or lymphoma. Prednisone remains the most commonly used treatment because most of these masses are due to lymphoma or leukemia. Other clues to the diagnosis may be apparent (organomegaly, generalized adenopathy, evidence of tumor lysis syndrome, elevated white blood cell [WBC] count, etc.). Hydration should be given and the child monitored for metabolic derangements that may be exacerbated by the initiation of therapy.

As an alternative to chemotherapy, radiation may be given, at 100 cGy in fractions for 1 to 4 days, with the goal of minimizing radiation scatter to the periphery of the tumor (preserve an area for biopsy and histologic evaluation) or the trachea. Tracheal swelling and airway compression can occur.

Continue evaluation and diagnostic studies when the patient is stable. The precise histologic diagnosis may not be possible following chemotherapy or radiation, even if the biopsy is done within 48 hours.

ABDOMINAL EMERGENCIES/TYPHLITIS

Abdominal emergencies in the child with cancer are usually related to the immune-compromised state and are a result of inflammation, mechanical obstruction, hemorrhage, or perforation. Effects of chemotherapy, malnutrition, underlying infections, and myelosuppression put these children at significant risk as a result of a blunted inflammatory response and poor wound healing.

EVALUATION

Children typically have abdominal pain, changes in vital signs (fever, hypo/hypertension, tachycardia); blood in the stool or emesis; abdominal distention, lack of bowel sounds (obstruction), or tinkles (ileus). The examination consists of observation, auscultation of the abdomen, palpation, and rectal exam only by an experienced person if absolutely necessary (risk of mucosal tear and introduction of infection with neutropenia).

DIAGNOSIS

Evaluate the patient for hemorrhage and infection (complete blood count with differential, blood culture, stool culture, electrolytes). Obtain plain radiographs (include decubitus views), a chest radiograph, and possibly a CT scan to evaluate for pneumatosis, bowel perforation, or presence and location of a mass. Direct visualization with endoscopy or colonoscopy may be necessary, but should be done cautiously in the setting of neutropenia. A barium swallow may be helpful to evaluate for esophagitis.

Typhlitis is defined as necrotizing enterocolitis localized to the cecum and typically occurs only in children with severe neutropenia. It may progress to bacterial invasion of the mucosa, inflammation, infarction, or perforation. *Clostridium septicum* and gram-negative bacteria (*Pseudomonas aeruginosa*) frequently are implicated. Typhlitis may be related to gastrointestinal tract (GI)–toxic chemotherapy that results in extensive mucositis.

Abdominal radiographs may demonstrate pneumatosis intestinalis, or nonspecific bowel wall thickening. CT may show thickening of the cecal wall and is highly suggestive in a patient with fever and neutropenia and right lower quadrant pain. The differential diagnosis includes pseudomembranous colitis and infection with *C. difficile*.

TREATMENT

Mortality is high (50% to 100%). Treatment consists of supportive care: fluids, pressors as necessary, broad-spectrum antibiotics to cover gram-negative and GI anaerobes, and hematologic (transfusion and cytokine) support.

Criteria for surgical intervention are persistent GI bleeding despite resolution of neutropenia, bleeding, free intraperitoneal air (perforation), clinical deterioration requiring vasopressor support and high-volume intravenous fluid (IVF) resuscitation (suggestive of uncontrolled sepsis from intestinal infarction), and development of a bowel obstruction. Pneumatosis and localized peritoneal signs are not sufficient to warrant surgical intervention.

HYPERLEUKOCYTOSIS

Hyperleukocytosis is defined as a peripheral WBC count exceeding 100,000/μl. It is most commonly seen at presentation or relapse of acute myelogenous leukemia (AML), acute lymphoblastic leukemia (ALL), or chronic myelogenous leukemia (CML). The incidence at presentation is

ALL: 9% to 13% of children at presentation
AML: 5% to 22% of children at presentation
CML: almost all children in the chronic phase

The risk of death increases greatly when the WBC count exceeds 300,000/μl. The most common complication seen with hyperleukocytosis is the tu-

20

HYPERLEUKOCYTOSIS

mor lysis syndrome. Central nervous system hemorrhage or thrombosis and pulmonary leukostasis are other potentially life-threatening complications. These problems are more commonly seen in AML because of the rheology of myeloblasts.

Hyperleukocytosis results in an increased blood viscosity by blast cell aggregates and thrombi in the microcirculation. Blasts have a large cell volume and are less deformable than normal WBCs, with a tendency to trap plasma. Viscosity is dependent on red cell and packed leukocyte volumes. Myeloblasts are large and adherent to each other and the vessel lumen (350 to 450 μm^3); lymphoblasts are smaller and nonadherent (250 to 350 μm^3). When the packed leukocyte volume is greater than 20% to 25%, the bulk viscosity of blood is increased.

Poor perfusion and anaerobic metabolism in the microcirculation lead to lactic acidosis. When WBC counts are greater than 300,000/μl, local proliferation of cells occurs within the cerebral vasculature and brain and vessel damage occurs, leading to secondary hemorrhage. Vessel damage can occur anywhere in the body, though the most clinically significant damage is in the brain and lungs.

EVALUATION

Signs and symptoms of leukemia are usually present (pallor, fatigue, fever, bleeding, or bone pain with adenopathy, organomegaly, anemia, and thrombocytopenia), with possible signs and symptoms of leukostasis in the lungs or brain (hypoxia, acidosis, dyspnea, cyanosis, blurred vision, papilledema, stupor, coma, or ataxia). Priapism may also occur in this setting.

The laboratory assessment should include frequent monitoring (q6–8h) of the WBC count to determine the rapidity of increase of the count or the response to therapy. Metabolic studies also need close monitoring because the child may have evidence of tumor lysis and renal dysfunction. Evaluate electrolytes, blood urea nitrogen (BUN), creatinine, uric acid, calcium, phosphorus, magnesium, liver function studies, and lactate dehydrogenase (LDH) at presentation, then monitor the lysis labs (electrolytes, calcium, phosphorus, magnesium, uric acid) and renal function studies (BUN, creatinine) frequently to assess response to therapy.

TREATMENT

Therapeutic intervention should be immediate. If the child is being transported, some simple measures should be initiated prior to transport. The mainstay of therapy is aggressive hydration, typically two to three times maintenance IVF with alkalinization (5% dextrose in water [D_5W] + 40 mEq sodium bicarbonate/L) to promote excretion of uric acid, and a hyperuricemic agent such as allopurinol or, preferably, urate oxidase (if available). If urate oxidase is given, alkalinization is usually not necessary because the uric acid falls precipitously, which then allows for better control of the hyperphosphatemia (tendency to precipitate in an alkaline pH).

If aggressive hydration does not bring the WBC count down quickly to 100,000 to 200,000/μl or the WBC count is rapidly rising because of rapid tumor growth, cytoreduction may be necessary. Leukapheresis and exchange transfusion are two methods that decrease tumor bulk, decrease the load on the kidneys, and can correct the anemia and hyperviscosity (>30% leukocyte reduction with a single leukapheresis). Exchange transfusion is more universally available, and it is recommended to begin with a single-volume exchange and perform diagnostic studies on the peripheral blood. Therapy for the underlying malignancy should begin as soon as possible and is the only permanent therapy for hyperleukocytosis. In general, it is safer from a metabolic viewpoint to initiate chemotherapy with a lower WBC count, following a cytoreductive technique. Cranial radiotherapy (400 cGy) is not currently recommended.

Transfusions should be given cautiously because of the potential to increase total blood viscosity and worsen leukostasis. Platelets can be given safely in small volumes because there are no cellular elements to increase the viscosity. Platelets should be given if the child is bleeding or the platelet count is less than 20×10^9/L. Red cell transfusions should be given with extreme caution, and only if the child is symptomatic of anemia or cardiovascularly compromised. The hemoglobin level should be kept below 10 g/dl.

TUMOR LYSIS SYNDROME

Tumor lysis syndrome is defined as the triad of hyperuricemia, hyperkalemia, and hyperphosphatemia. It is often complicated by secondary renal failure and symptomatic hypocalcemia.

Children with tumors of high growth rate present with tumor lysis or frequently develop it within the first 5 days of treatment. Their tumors are usually exquisitely sensitive to chemotherapy. Standard-risk ALL and nonlymphomatous solid tumors do not usually present in this manner. High-risk ALL (high WBC count) and advanced-stage lymphomas (classically Burkitt's lymphoma) present with a large tumor mass, high doubling time (38 to 116 hours in Burkitt's lymphoma), poor urine output, and elevated uric acid and LDH.

Tumor lysis syndrome is a direct result of degradation of malignant cells and inadequate renal function. Uric acid, potassium, and phosphorus are excreted by the kidney. Elevated uric acid is a result of the breakdown of nucleic acids, which can precipitate in the collecting ducts in the acid environment of the kidney. Lactic acidosis, secondary to poor tissue oxygenation in patients with high WBC counts, may contribute to uric acid deposition. Phosphates are released when tumor cells lyse. When the calcium–phosphorus product exceeds 60, precipitates occur in the microvasculature, particularly in an alkaline environment. This may lead to renal failure. Lymphoblasts are rich in phosphate (four times the level in normal lymphocytes). Hypocalcemia and seizures can also occur secondary to hyperphosphatemia. Potassium is also released from tumor cells, and is secondarily elevated in poor renal function, and can lead to fatal arrhythmia.

EVALUATION

Evaluate the patient for signs and symptoms of metabolic abnormalities. Perform a metabolic panel in all children with suspected malignancy to assess for tumor lysis. The tumor lysis syndrome should be constantly assessed for early in therapy as well, particularly in patients with high tumor burdens and who are expected to respond rapidly to treatment.

Assess electrolytes, calcium, magnesium, phosphorus, uric acid, LDH, BUN, and creatinine at time of presentation and q4–8h dependent on the underlying disease, initiation of therapy, and risk for tumor lysis syndrome.

Evaluate vital signs, urine output (evidence of renal failure), and possible symptoms of hypocalcemia (anorexia, vomiting, cramps, spasms, tetany, and seizures). A renal ultrasound may be indicated in suspected renal dysfunction.

THERAPY

Aggressive hydration with alkalinization and hyperuricemic agents should be initiated immediately. Allopurinol (or urate oxidase, if available) can be given at presentation and as needed during the early phase of therapy for the prevention or treatment of hyperuricemia. Urate oxidase is a recombinant enzyme that acts as a catalyst in the degradation of uric acid into allantoin, a highly soluble product compared to uric acid. It works quickly (within 30 minutes of IV infusion) and keeps the uric acid level low for 12 to 24 hours or longer, depending on the underlying rate of cell turnover. Urate oxidase has been studied in children with cancer who have hyperuricemia as a result of tumor lysis and has been found to be safe and effective. It is currently awaiting Food and Drug Administration approval, but is available on a compassionate use basis. IVF should not contain potassium until it can be determined that the patient's potassium level is stable and not increasing as a result of tumor lysis or renal insufficiency. Maintain a urine pH of 7.0 to 7.5 to promote uric acid excretion (not necessary with the use of urate oxidase).

Other therapeutic steps include the following:

- Hydration: provide two to three times maintenance IVF with D_5W + 40 mEq/L sodium bicarbonate (titrate bicarbonate to as high as 80 mEq/L to maintain alkaline urine pH of 7.0 to 7.5).
- Give allopurinol 300 mg/m^2/day divided q8h (800 mg/day maximum) or urate oxidase 0.2 mg/kg/day in 50 ml preservative-free normal saline IV over 30 minutes.
- Ensure adequate urine output (balanced intake and output, taking into account insensible losses).
- Institute frequent metabolic monitoring (q4–8h).

Obtain a cardiac echocardiogram and electrocardiogram (ECG) if the potassium is 6 mEq/L or higher. The ECG may show wide QRS complexes and peaked T waves in hyperkalemia.

Hyperkalemia may require therapy with Kayexalate, calcium gluconate, or insulin. If hyperphosphatemia is present, treatment is with ALternaGEL and decreasing urine alkalinization.

SUGGESTED READING

Albano EA, Ablin AR. Oncologic emergencies. In: Ablin AR (ed), Supportive Care of Children with Cancer, 2nd ed. Baltimore: The Johns Hopkins University Press, 1997, pp 175–192.

Lange B, O'Neill JA, Goldwein JW, et al. Oncologic emergencies. In: Pizzo PA, Poplack DG (eds), Principles and Practice of Pediatric Oncology, 3rd ed. Philadelphia: Lippincott–Raven, 1997, pp 1025–1050.

Pui CH, Mahmoud HH, Wiley JM, et al. Recombinant urate oxidase for the prophylaxis or treatment of hyperuricemia in patients with leukemia or lymphoma. J Clin Oncol 19:697–704, 2001.

20

TUMOR LYSIS SYNDROME

ACUTE LEUKEMIA

21

ACUTE LYMPHOBLASTIC LEUKEMIA

Acute leukemia is the most common type of cancer in children, with an incidence of 3 to 4 cases per 100,000 Caucasian children each year in the United States. Approximately 2500 to 3000 new cases are diagnosed each year in this country. The peak incidence is between 2 and 5 years of age. Overall, acute leukemia accounts for approximately 30% of childhood cancer cases. Acute lymphocytic leukemia (ALL) accounts for 75% of the total number of cases of acute leukemia, followed by acute myeloid leukemia (AML) in 20%, followed by other rarer forms.

The etiology of acute leukemia is unknown, but many predisposing genetic, environmental, and viral factors have been implicated. Ionizing radiation and exposure to benzene have been associated with an increased risk of developing leukemia. Certain syndromes and chromosomal abnormalities have also been associated with a high incidence of developing leukemia (Down syndrome, Fanconi's anemia, Bloom syndrome, ataxia–telangiectasia). Siblings, in particular identical twins, have an increased risk of developing leukemia as children. Most cases of leukemia stem from somatic genetic alterations, as opposed to an inherited genetic predisposition.

The acute leukemias are biologically classified by blast morphology, surface proteins, cytogenetic abnormalities, and cytochemical staining. This information, in addition to clinical features, is important in stratifying groups of children by type of leukemia and risk group. Therapy is risk based, with the goal of providing optimal curative potential while minimizing risks and side effects. Most cases of ALL arise from B-cell–committed progenitors. Children with T-cell ALL tend to have other high-risk features, such as older age (over 10 years), initial high white blood cell (WBC) count, and lymphomatous features (massive adenopathy, organomegaly, mediastinal mass). The outcome is best for those with early pre-B-cell ALL, intermediate for those with pre-B-cell or T-cell ALL, and worst for those with B-cell ALL. Cytogenetic abnormalities are common and also provide prognostic information. Hyperdiploidy is associated with a favorable outcome, whereas certain translocations such as t(9:22), t(4:11), and t(1:19) are associated with poorer outcomes.

CLINICAL PRESENTATION

The clinical manifestations of leukemia are a direct result of the marrow invasion and resultant cytopenias (anemia, thrombocytopenia, leukopenia and/or neutropenia) and extramedullary involvement. Children with anemia may have pallor, fatigue, tachycardia, or evidence of congestive heart failure. Infection may be present at diagnosis, causing fever, likely secondary to neutropenia. Bleeding is usually mild and manifested as petechiae, bruising, gingival oozing, or epistaxis. Life-threatening hemorrhage may occur, but is very rare. Lymphadenopathy or a mediastinal mass may be extensive, resulting in airway or cardiovascular compromise (see Chapter 20).

Central nervous system (CNS) involvement occurs in approximately 5% of children at presentation. The majority of patients are asymptomatic, though there may be signs and symptoms of increased intracranial pressure (cranial nerve VI palsy, morning headache, vomiting, papilledema). Rarely, there may be signs or symptoms of parenchymal involvement, hypothalamic syndrome, or diabetes insipidus. Other rare complications, such as chloromas causing compression of the spinal cord or CNS hemorrhage (related to leukostasis, coagulopathy), are more likely to be associated with AML.

Leukemic involvement of the **testes** occurs in 2% to 5% of boys at presentation and presents as painless enlargement of the testes, either bilateral or unilateral. Early testicular involvement is also associated with other high-risk factors such as T-cell disease, elevated WBC count, and lymphomatous features.

Bone pain is present in approximately 25% of children at diagnosis (Table 21–1). In very young children, the initial symptoms are irritability and refusal to walk. This may result from direct leukemic infiltration of the periosteum, or expansion of the marrow cavity by leukemic cells. Pathologic fractures may also be present at diagnosis and cause significant pain.

Radiographic changes of the bones are common and include

- Osteolytic lesions involving the medullary cavity or cortex
- Subperiosteal new bone formation
- Pathologic fracture
- Transverse metaphyseal radiolucent bands
- Transverse metaphyseal lines of increased density (growth arrest lines)

TABLE 21–1
COMMON CLINICAL AND LABORATORY FEATURES OF ALL AT PRESENTATION

FINDING	PERCENTAGE OF PATIENTS
Fever	60
Pallor	40
Bleeding	50
Bone pain	25
Lymphadenopathy	50
Splenomegaly	60
Hepatosplenomegaly	70
White blood cell count (μl)	
<10,000	50
10,000–49,000	30
≥50,000	20
Hemoglobin (g/dl)	
<7.0	40
7.0–11.0	45
>11.0	15
Platelet count (μl)	
<20,000	30
20,000–99,000	45
≥100,000	25

DIAGNOSTIC STUDIES

When the diagnosis of leukemia is suspected based on the history, physical, or preliminary laboratory results (cytopenias, blasts identified on a peripheral smear), the following laboratory studies are indicated:

- Complete blood count, differential, review of peripheral blood smear
- Bone marrow aspirate (consider biopsy for dry tap or inadequate specimen) for morphology, blast count, immunophenotyping, cytogenetics, cytochemistry
- Metabolic panel, to include liver function studies, electrolytes, lactate dehydrogenase, uric acid, phosphorus, calcium, blood urea nitrogen, creatinine
- Coagulation profile (prothrombin time, activated partial thromboplastin time, fibrinogen, D-dimers of fibrin degradation products)
- Blood culture if febrile, cultures of other suspected sites of infection

Additionally, a chest radiograph should be obtained to evaluate for the possible presence of a mediastinal mass.

Typically, the bone marrow is 80% to 100% replaced at the time of diagnosis. At times, because of the packed condition of the marrow, it may be difficult to aspirate a sample (dry tap). The diagnosis of acute leukemia requires the presence of 25% or more blasts in the marrow; however, the diagnosis is suspect when the marrow contains more than 5%. After the diagnosis of leukemia is confirmed by the above studies (and type of leukemia as well), further studies prior to therapy may include the following:

1. Viral serologies are done for hepatitis B and C, cytomegalovirus, herpes simplex virus, and varicella zoster virus (baseline information prior to transfusion and/or in the event of an exposure to one of these infectious agents so as to provide information with regard to passive immunization or therapy).
2. A lumbar puncture is done to assess possible involvement of the cerebrospinal fluid (CSF) and to assist with therapeutic decisions and classification. A cell count and cytocentrifuge examination for cell morphology is done on the fresh CSF. The diagnosis of CNS leukemia requires the presence of 5 or more WBCs/μl and identification of blasts on the CSF cytocentrifuge examination. CNS leukemia is classified as follows:
   a. CNS1: less than 5 WBCs/μl, no blasts
   b. CNS2: less than 5 WBCs/μl, blasts present
   c. CNS3: 5 or more WBCs/μl and blasts present
3. Quantitative immunoglobulins and complement levels should be determined.
4. Echocardiogram and electrocardiogram should be done, especially if induction therapy includes an anthracycline (cardiac toxic).

RISK GROUP CLASSIFICATION

Patients are stratified into treatment groups based on age and WBC count at the time of presentation. Further stratification is done within the first few weeks of therapy and is dependent on early response to therapy (as measured by the results of the day 7 and/or day 14 bone marrow aspirate), cytogenetic abnormalities identified on the diagnostic marrow, and remission status at the end of induction. Other considerations include immunophenotype and presence of CNS disease.

Patients fall into the **standard-risk** group if the age is between 1 and 9 years and the presenting WBC count is less than 50,000/μl. Children 10 years of age and older and those with a WBC count of 50,000/μl or higher are automatically considered **high risk** and treated more aggressively. Infants have a special category and are a particularly high-risk group, especially the very young infant. Children who have high-risk features identified after initial diagnosis (high-risk translocations, poor response to therapy) may be selectively diverted to receive more aggressive therapy. Patients with T-cell disease or the presence of lymphomatous features are believed by some investigators to be at higher risk and may also be treated more aggressively than patients without these features.

TREATMENT

The purpose of therapy is to induce a biologic and clinical remission (no evidence of disease on laboratory and physical assessment). Overall, 65% to 75% of children with leukemia will be cured of their disease with modern combination chemotherapy. Treatment regimens are divided into phases of therapy:

- **Induction:** refers to first 28 to 35 days of therapy, after which the child should be in remission. Remission induction rate in standard-risk ALL is 98%.
- **Consolidation:** further chemotherapy is given, in addition to a focus on CNS prophylaxis.
- **Interim maintenance**
- **Delayed intensification:** refers to reinduction and reconsolidation; may be given once or twice, dependent on the protocol.
- **Maintenance:** continuation of therapy; this phase lasts 2 to 3 years.

Conventional induction therapy includes prednisone or dexamethasone, asparaginase, and vincristine. High-risk patients also receive doxorubicin. Additional drugs such as cyclophosphamide, cytarabine, 6-thioguanine, and anthracyclines are added in the delayed intensification phase of the therapy and have significantly improved the outcome in most patients. Maintenance consists of pulses of steroid (prednisone or dexamethasone) and vincristine in addition to methotrexate and 6-mercaptopurine. CNS prophylaxis is provided by means of intrathecal chemotherapy, either methotrexate alone or triple drugs (methotrexate, hydrocortisone, and cytarabine). Children who present with CNS3 disease traditionally receive augmented therapy with 1800 cGy cranial radiation, in addition to intrathecal chemotherapy. Some centers also advocate treating children with CNS2 disease more aggressively as well. Without CNS prophylaxis, it is estimated that 60% to 70% of children would relapse in the CNS (based on historical data).

Most children with cancer in the United States are treated at pediatric oncology centers and have access to participation in clinical trials. These studies have accelerated the advances made in the diagnosis and treatment of pediatric cancer and clearly are a major reason for many of the successes. The Children's Oncology Group (COG) is a national collaborative group of professionals involved in the treatment of children with cancer. Most pediatric cancer centers register patients in these trials, follow the protocols, and submit data. Families are asked to give informed consent to participate in these trials, which may include clinical and biologic questions. For families not wishing to participate, the existing standard of care is offered (best published information on treatment of the specific malignancy). Many centers may also participate in smaller pilot studies or have their own protocols.

COMPLICATIONS OF THERAPY

Because of the myelosuppressive nature of the therapy and the underlying disease state, children undergoing chemotherapy or radiation may expect to have complications during the course of their therapy. Many of these complications can be predicted and prevented. Most patients will require transfusion support with packed red blood cells and/or platelets. Children with neutropenia need to take special precautions to decrease the risk of infection exposure. Any child receiving chemotherapy who develops a fever should have emergent medical attention, especially during phases of anticipated neutropenia (induction, consolidation, delayed intensification). Some therapies may be neurotoxic (vincristine, intrathecal therapy, radiation), and children should be monitored for these toxicities (see Chapters 17 and 20).

RELAPSE

Approximately 25% to 35% of children with ALL may experience a relapse, most commonly in the bone marrow or in extramedullary sites such as the CNS and testes. The timing of relapse is critical; in general the earlier the relapse (<18 months in remission) the worse the prognosis. Depending on the site and timing of relapse, bone marrow transplantation (BMT) may be offered as therapy, following successful re-induction chemotherapy. Overall survival for relapse is 40% to 50%, partly because of cumulative toxicity from prior therapy and high infection rates. In general, children with late, isolated extramedullary relapse fare better. Early bone marrow relapse has a particularly poor prognosis, irrespective of treatment.

ACUTE MYELOGENOUS LEUKEMIA

AML accounts for about 20% to 25% of all acute leukemias in childhood that are nonlymphoblastic. It represents a heterogeneous group of disorders classified morphologically and cytochemically as M0 through M7 (Table 21–2). AML has a constant incidence from birth through adolescence without a clear age peak. In general, the prognosis for AML is poorer than that for ALL, with long-term survivals of 50% to 60%.

The etiology for AML is not known, but there is an increased incidence in children with certain genetic disorders such as Down, Fanconi's, Kostmann's, Bloom and Diamond-Blackfan syndromes. Children who develop second malignancies (some related to prior therapy) tend to develop AML. Those with myeloproliferative or myelodysplastic disease also have a predisposition to developing AML.

Some classical chromosomal abnormalities are seen in AML and may help determine a more precise diagnosis or portend prognostic significance. The t(8;21) (22q,11q) translocation is the most common chromosome translocation and is associated with a more favorable prognosis. The t(15; 17) (22q,11q) translocation is classically seen in acute promyeloblastic leukemia (APL) (M3), and inversion of chromosome 16 is associated with acute myelomonoblastic leukemia (M4). Monosomy 7 is associated with secondary malignancies and myeloproliferative disorders and is particularly difficult to treat successfully. M7 is also classically associated with Down syndrome. Myelomonocytic, monocytic, erythroid, and megakaryoblastic subtypes are associated with poorer prognoses.

CLINICAL PRESENTATION

AML presents in a fashion similar to ALL and frequently is indistinguishable at presentation. The most common clinical symptom is fever, occurring in 70% of patients at initial diagnosis. Symptoms of the cytopenias may be evident, with pallor, fatigue, anorexia, and bleeding. Gingival hypertrophy is a clinical feature highly suggestive of AML. Adenopathy may be present, but

TABLE 21–2
MORPHOLOGIC CLASSIFICATION FOR AML

M0	Undifferentiated leukemia
M1	Acute myeloblastic leukemia without differentiation
M2	Acute myeloblastic leukemia with differentiation
M3	Acute promyeloblastic leukemia
M4	Acute myelomonoblastic leukemia
M5	Acute monocytic leukemia
M6	Erythroleukemia
M7	Acute megakaryoblastic leukemia

in general is not as bulky as can be seen in ALL. Chloromas (extramedullary collections of blast cells) are sometimes seen in patients with AML and may present as subcutaneous, nontender masses. Infants may have subcutaneous nodules.

LABORATORY EVALUATION
The same studies suggested for the evaluation of ALL should be obtained in the evaluation of the child with suspected AML. It is common to see severe anemia and thrombocytopenia in association with an elevated total WBC count. Children with extreme leukocytosis (over 200,000 to 300,000/μl) may present with metabolic abnormalities and tumor lysis syndrome. Clinically they are at risk for hypoxia in the small vessels of the brain and lungs as a result of the increased viscosity of the blood because of the presence of large, adherent myeloblasts. Abnormal coagulation studies may be seen, with evidence of overt disseminated intravascular coagulation in children with extreme hyperleukocytosis or APL. In APL, the coagulation abnormality is thought to be due to tissue thromboplastin activity from the intracellular granules. The definitive diagnosis is made with evaluation of the bone marrow, with at least 25% to 30% of the cellular elements being myeloblasts. Identification of the cell lineage is confirmed by immunophenotyping and cytochemistry. Cytogenetic studies are also performed on the marrow. A lumbar puncture should be done; up to 5% of children will have overt involvement of the CSF.

RISK GROUP CLASSIFICATION
Though certain factors are associated with a lower remission rate, all children with AML, with the exception of those with APL and children with Down syndrome, are treated in a similar fashion. Poor risk features include presenting WBC count over 100,000/μl, monosomy 7, and secondary AML. Good risk features include M1 or M2 with Auer rods, M3, or M4; rapid response to initial therapy; Down syndrome; and favorable chromosomal abnormalities, such as t(8;21), t(15;17), and inversion 16.

TREATMENT
The therapy necessary to induce remission and provide long-term control or cure is more intensive and toxic as compared to the therapy for ALL. As with ALL, the goal of induction therapy is to induce a clinical and biologic remission by elimination of the malignant cell line. Approximately 80% of children achieve remission with induction therapy. The most effective induction regimens include daunomycin, cytarabine, etoposide, dexamethasone, and 6-thioguanine. Allogeneic BMT is recommended for all patients who have a suitable family human lymphocyte antigen–matched donor and achieve remission status. In the absence of such a donor, the patient should be treated with intensive chemotherapy to include cytarabine and asparaginase in addition to the above-mentioned regimen. CNS con-

solidative therapy with intrathecal cytarabine is also included in the treatment plan. Children with Down syndrome have a particularly favorable prognosis and receive chemotherapy only in a less intensive manner. Overall, children with AML (not including APL) who receive an allogeneic BMT have an expected survival of 65%.

Children with APL have a particularly good prognosis and receive treatment that includes all-*trans* retinoic acid (ATRA). ATRA is associated with the differentiation of immature promyelocytes into mature granulocytes, followed by restoration of normal hematopoiesis. ATRA does not cross the blood–brain barrier and is therefore ineffective in treating CNS involvement with APL. These children should also receive cytarabine and an anthracycline as part of their treatment. Studies investigating arsenic as a differentiation agent are also being conducted in this disease.

COMPLICATIONS OF THERAPY

Given the intensity of the therapy for AML, children can expect to experience a number of complications, which include intensive blood product support, mucositis, liver toxicity, and severe marrow suppression. Infection is common and should be monitored for closely. These children are a particularly high risk for development of sepsis with gram-negative organisms in addition to invasive fungal disease. *Streptococcus viridans* sepsis is associated with the use of high-dose cytarabine and resultant altered integrity of the gastrointestinal mucosa. Sepsis with this organism can be rapidly fatal. Many institutions treat children receiving AML therapy with prophylactic antibiotics and antifungal agents. Empiric therapy for fever and neutropenia should include coverage for *S. viridans* and be started immediately with a first fever.

Coagulopathy at diagnosis is not uncommon, especially in the child with APL. Surveillance studies should be done routinely and coagulopathies treated as appropriate to maintain fibrinogen levels above 100 mg/dl and platelet counts above 20,000 to 50,000/μl.

Prolonged hospitalization is expected during the course of treatment for AML. These patients should be in protective environments and frequently need parenteral nutrition, antibiotics, and blood product support for most of the treatment period.

RELAPSE

The prognosis for children who are refractory to initial therapy or who relapse is very poor. Chemotherapy alone results in less than 10% 1-year disease-free survival, whereas BMT (allogeneic or unrelated fully matched) may improve outcome to 30% to 50%.

SUGGESTED READING

Diamond CA. Oncology. In: Rudolph AM, Kamei RK (eds), Rudolph's Fundamentals of Pediatrics, 2nd ed. Norwalk, CT: Appleton & Lange, 1998, pp 491–510.

Golub TR, Weinstein HJ, Grier HE. Acute myelogenous leukemia. In: Pizzo PA, Poplack DG (eds), Principles and Practice of Pediatric Oncology, 3rd ed. Philadelphia: Lippincott–Raven, 1997, pp 463–482.

Margolin JF, Poplack DG. Acute lymphoblastic leukemia. In: Pizzo PA, Poplack DG (eds), Principles and Practice of Pediatric Oncology, 3rd ed. Philadelphia: Lippincott–Raven, 1997, pp 409–462.

CENTRAL NERVOUS SYSTEM TUMORS

Brain tumors are the second most common group of malignant tumors, accounting for 20% of all childhood malignancies. The most common location is infratentorial, with medulloblastomas, astrocytomas, and meningiomas occurring in the cerebellum and astrocytomas, ependymomas, and glioblastomas occurring in the brain stem. Approximately 40% of tumors are supratentorial in location, with astrocytomas, ependymomas, glioblastomas, and meningiomas occurring in the cerebral hemispheres. Tumors specific to the sella or chiasm are craniopharyngiomas, pituitary adenomas, and optic nerve gliomas.

The majority of brain tumors are sporadic, though a small percentage are associated with genetic disorders such as neurofibromatosis, tuberous sclerosis, von Hippel–Lindau syndrome, and Li-Fraumeni syndrome (germline mutation of p53, a suppressor oncogene). Brain tumors may also occur as second malignancies in children previously treated for leukemia or with central nervous system (CNS) radiation. Some chromosomal abnormalities have been identified in pediatric brain tumors and may be useful in pathologic classification. In general, brain tumor classification is based on embryonic derivation and histologic cell of origin. Microscopic criteria useful in grading of tumors include cellular pleomorphism, mitotic index, anaplasia, and necrosis.

CLINICAL PRESENTATION

Signs and symptoms of **intracranial** brain tumors are related to the location and rate of tumor growth. The most common presenting signs and symptoms are related to increased intracranial pressure (ICP) or focal neurologic deficits. Children may present with headache, irritability, vomiting, focal seizures, ataxia, cranial neuropathies, visual field defects, papilledema, Parinaud syndrome (failure of upward gaze and setting-sun sign), endocrine abnormalities, or diencephalic syndrome (failure to thrive and emaciation).

CNS tumors may also occur anywhere along the vertebral column. **Spinal tumors** cause symptoms as a result of compression of the spinal canal. The most common symptom is back pain, a distinctly unusual complaint in children and adolescents. The pain is worse in the supine position or with Valsalva's maneuver. Spinal tumors may occur in the intramedullary space (glial tumors such as astrocytomas, ependymomas, and oligodendrogliomas). Tumors in the extramedullary compartment are either intradural or extradural. Intradural tumors are most likely to be neurofibromas or meningiomas. Extradural tumors tend to be of mesenchymal origin, often a direct extension of a tumor into the intervertebral foramina. Neuroblastoma and lymphomas may present with spinal cord extension. Tumors in the vertebral bodies (histiocytosis, primary bone tumors,

tumors metastatic to bone) can cause epidural compression and resultant paraplegia.

DIAGNOSTIC EVALUATION

RADIOGRAPHIC IMAGING

Computed tomography (CT) scans of the brain, with and without contrast, should be performed in a child with a suspected intracranial tumor. CT is more useful than **magnetic resonance imaging** (MRI) in evaluating bony lesions, detecting tumor calcifications, and imaging unstable patients because of its shorter imaging time and greater local availability. In many centers, MRI with gadolinium–diethylenetriaminepenta-acetic acid (Gd-DTPA) is becoming the preferred diagnostic evaluation, especially in the preoperative setting. It provides greater sensitivity in areas that may be obscured by proximity to bone, such as the temporal lobe and posterior fossa. MRI also provides multiplanar images. Contrast MRI allows for identification of tumor within areas of surrounding edema, detects focal areas of blood–brain barrier breakdown, and improves delineation of cysts from solid tumor.

Positron emission tomography (PET) is a potentially useful technique for evaluating CNS tumors. Metabolic differences between normal tissue and malignant tumor can be detected with the ^{18}F-labeled analogue of 2-deoxyglucose. Astrocytomas and oligodendrogliomas are hypometabolic and anaplastic astrocytomas and glioblastoma multiforme are hypermetabolic. PET may be useful in determining the degree of tumor aggressiveness and appropriate biopsy site; differentiating recurrent tumor from necrosis, scar, and edema in the postoperative period; or following therapy with chemotherapy or radiation.

Spinal cord tumors should be imaged with MRI with Gd-DTPA. Myelography is not routinely used. Patients with intracranial tumors with the potential to metastasize to the spinal cord should have a spinal MRI, though this may be done after a pathologic diagnosis is confirmed.

ADDITIONAL STUDIES

A **lumbar puncture** with evaluation of the cerebrospinal fluid (CSF) should be performed in children with tumors in close proximity to the circulating CSF or those with the potential to metastasize to the CSF (medulloblastoma, ependymoma, and brain stem gliomas). A cell count (white cells, red cells), glucose, protein, and cytocentrifuge to identify possible malignant cells should be performed on the CSF. **CSF tumor markers** (α-fetoprotein and human chorionic gonadotropin) may be elevated in CNS germ cell tumors.

A **bone marrow aspirate** is indicated in children with confirmed medulloblastoma or high-grade ependymomas because these tumors do have the potential for systemic metastasis. A **bone scan** may also be indicated in these situations.

TREATMENT

Therapies offered to children with brain tumors are dependent on the histology, location, resectability, and prognosis related to the individual tumor. Modalities for therapy include surgery, radiation, and chemotherapy. **Neurosurgical intervention** is indicated in the majority of patients (excluding intrinsic brain stem tumors). The goals of neurosurgical intervention are to attempt maximum tumor removal with low morbidity and mortality, attain tissue for a histologic diagnosis, and possibly relieve CSF obstruction and resultant ICP by tumor debulking and/or placement of a ventricular shunt.

Most children with brain tumors require **radiation therapy** because of incomplete surgical resection and high likelihood of tumor regrowth. The dose of radiation is dependent on the type of tumor, age of the child, and location and volume to be irradiated. In young children (under age 5 years), it can be expected that there will be significant impairment of intellectual and physical development as a result of this therapy. Newer strategies continue to be developed to avoid or delay radiation in very young children with CNS tumors.

Until recently, **chemotherapy** was not used in the adjuvant setting in the treatment of primary CNS tumors. The blood–brain barrier was thought to prevent adequate penetration of tumor with effective concentrations of chemotherapeutic agents. However, it is apparent that many drugs do adequately cross into the CSF. Other factors, such as tumor heterogeneity, cell kinetics, drug distribution, and drug excretion, may have a more significant impact on effectiveness of therapy. Tumors with a low mitotic index and slow growth are less sensitive to chemotherapy; tumors with a high mitotic index and high growth rate are more sensitive to chemotherapy. Intrathecal chemotherapy is often also given in cases of meningeal spread or in those tumors for which the risk of spread to the CSF is high. Commonly used drugs for the treatment of brain tumors include vincristine, methotrexate, procarbazine, carmustine (BCNU), lomustine (CCNU), cisplatin, carboplatin, etoposide, and prednisone.

MEDULLOBLASTOMAS

Medulloblastomas are also known as primitive neuroectodermal tumors and are the most common CNS tumor in children, accounting for 20% to 30% of all childhood brain tumors. They typically present in the posterior fossa and, in up to 40% of cases at diagnosis, widespread seeding of the subarachnoid space or to areas outside the CNS may occur. Increased ICP may be present as a result of obstruction of the fourth ventricle. Ventricular shunting may be necessary preoperatively, and a Millipore filter should be placed to decrease or prevent the flow of tumor cells in the spinal fluid.

Staging studies should follow initial imaging of the brain and histologic confirmation of the tumor. Other studies should include an MRI of the

22

MEDULLOBLASTOMAS

spine, CSF cytology, skeletal survey, chest radiograph, and bone marrow evaluation. Tumor size, degree of resection, local extension, and presence of metastases are used in assessing prognosis and determination of therapy. Average-risk features are negative CSF cytology, negative spine MRI, Chang stages T1 or T2 (tumor less than 3 cm and at most invading one adjacent structure or partially filling the fourth ventricle), and over 4 years of age at diagnosis. Positive CSF cytology, positive spine MRI, advanced Chang stage (large tumor size and/or further invasion of CNS structures), focal differentiation on histology, or age less than 4 years at diagnosis are high-risk features.

Surgical excision is the initial therapy. Children with radical resections have a distinct survival advantage. Medulloblastomas are very radiosensitive, and radiation is a mainstay of therapy. Radiation in the child under 3 years of age is controversial because of the devastating long-term consequences on brain growth. Chemotherapy should be utilized to postpone or possibly avoid the use of high doses of radiation. In patients with high-risk features, chemotherapy is recommended after completion of craniospinal radiation. Average-risk patients also benefit from adjuvant chemotherapy following surgery and craniospinal radiation. Typical drug regimens incorporate vincristine, CCNU, prednisone, and cisplatin. Autologous bone marrow transplantation is being investigated for high-risk patients with poor initial response to therapy.

Five-year survival for children with average-risk medulloblastoma treated with surgery and radiation alone is 60% to 80%. This survival may be increased to 90% with adjuvant chemotherapy in some groups of patients. High-risk patients have a disease-free survival of 20% to 40% at 5 years with surgery and radiation alone, and up to 45% to 50% with adjuvant chemotherapy.

ASTROCYTOMAS

Cerebellar astrocytomas account for between 10% and 20% of CNS tumors and typically occur in the young child, less than 10 years of age. Most of these tumors are confined to the cerebellum and rarely progress to involve the neuraxis. Cerebral astrocytomas tend to be high grade and more infiltrative in nature. Histologically, astrocytomas are divided into low grade and high grade based on cellular pleomorphism, cell density, mitotic index, and necrosis. Low-grade astrocytomas typically are very slow growing and may present at a large size with symptoms such as seizures, focal neurologic deficits, or clinical evidence of hydrocephalus.

Surgical excision is the treatment of choice for astrocytomas. If removal is complete, no further treatment is necessary. In patients with residual tumor, radiation is recommended. The typical dose of radiation is 5400 to 5500 cGy in the child over age 5 years. In the very young child, it is possible that chemotherapy may allow for avoidance of or delay in radiation therapy. A current study is evaluating the role of chemotherapy (carboplatin, vincristine) in this setting. Children with partially resected low-grade tumors receiving postoperative radiation have a survival rate at 5 and 10 years of 50% and 25%, respectively.

Pilocytic cerebellar astrocytomas tend to be slow growing and are usually low grade. The majority of these tumors are amenable to complete resection, and patients have a very high survival rate (90% 10-year survival). If only partial resection is possible, then radiation is recommended and may improve survival. Postoperative radiation significantly improves the 5-year survival in partially resected cases from 35% to 50% with surgery alone to 80% with surgery and radiation. The use of chemotherapy in the adjuvant setting is limited and is not typically recommended.

In children with high-grade astrocytomas, surgical removal is rarely accomplished. However, surgical debulking reduces tumor burden and can prolong survival. Postoperative radiation is recommended. The dose is high, typically 5000 to 6000 cGy. Adjuvant chemotherapy following radiation has resulted in improved survival compared with radiation alone. Chemotherapy drugs that have activity in this disease include thiotepa, etoposide, BCNU, CCNU, vincristine, and prednisone.

EPENDYMOMAS

Ependymomas represent approximately 5% to 10% of all primary brain tumors in childhood. The fourth ventricle is the most common location, though these tumors may arise infratentorially or supratentorially. Ependymomas can also occur in the spinal cord and account for 25% of spinal tumors. The most common presenting problem is hydrocephalus. Surgical resection is often attempted, though complete removal of these tumors is rarely accomplished. Postoperative radiation has resulted in a significant improvement in survival rates. Subarachnoid dissemination may occur in these tumors; therefore, the spine should be imaged with MRI and the CSF cytology should be reviewed. Craniospinal radiation is given in doses of 4500 to 5000 cGy to the primary tumor and 3000 to 3500 cGy to the spine. Spinal radiation is given to children with high-grade posterior fossa and supratentorial tumors. Adjuvant chemotherapy is given with radiation (weekly vincristine for 6 doses) and postradiation. Vincristine, platinum agents, CCNU, and etoposide are agents with activity against this tumor.

The prognosis of a child with ependymoma is dependent on the grade of the tumor, resectability, and response to therapy. Low-grade tumors have a 5-year survival of 70%, while high-grade tumors have a poor survival of 15% to 20% at 5 years.

SUGGESTED READING

Heideman RL, Packer RJ, Albright AL, et al. Tumors of the central nervous system. In: Pizzo PA, Polack DG (eds), Principles and Practice of Pediatric Oncology, 3rd ed. Philadelphia: Lippincott–Raven, 1997, pp 633–698.

Lanzkowsky P. Manual of Pediatric Hematology and Oncology, 3rd ed. San Diego: Academic Press, 2000.

HODGKIN'S AND NON-HODGKIN'S LYMPHOMAS

Hodgkin's and non-Hodgkin's lymphomas together account for approximately 10% to 12% of malignancies in children; they are third in relative frequency after acute leukemias and brain tumors. Non-Hodgkin's lymphomas (NHLs) comprise approximately 60% of all lymphomas.

23

HODGKIN'S DISEASE

There is a bimodal distribution of cases of Hodgkin's disease, with a peak in adolescence to early adulthood (15 to 34 years) and a second peak in older adults (55 to 74 years). Overall, the incidence has slight male predominance. Hodgkin's disease is rarely diagnosed in children younger than 5 years of age. There is an increased incidence among siblings and family members. There is no clear association with congenital syndromes, though it has been reported in association with systemic lupus erythematosus, rheumatoid arthritis, ataxia–telangiectasia, agammaglobulinemia, human immunodeficiency virus (HIV), and Epstein-Barr virus (EBV). It is a disease seen more commonly in Caucasians and in those of higher socioeconomic status.

Several epidemiologic studies have suggested that infectious agents may be involved in the transmission of Hodgkin's disease. These agents include herpesvirus 6, cytomegalovirus, and EBV. Many patients have high EBV titers at diagnosis, suggesting that enhanced activation may precede the development of Hodgkin's disease. This hypothesis is supported by evidence of EBV genomes in Reed-Sternberg cells. The etiology of Hodgkin's disease, like other childhood malignancies, is complex and involves genetics, environmental factors, and possibly some degree of immune incompetence leading to poor immune surveillance and susceptibility to developing a malignancy.

The presumed malignant cell in Hodgkin's disease is the Reed-Sternberg cell, though these cells account for less than 1% of the involved tissue. These cells have the appearance of owl eyes on light microscopy. They have two or more nuclei or nuclear lobes and two or more large, inclusion-like nucleoli. Lacunar cell variants of the Reed-Sternberg cell are present in two histologic categories, the nodular sclerosing type and the nodular variant of lymphocyte-predominant Hodgkin's disease. The origin of the Reed-Sternberg cell is not yet determined but it may be from a T- or B-cell lineage. These cells occur singly or in clusters, surrounded by stromal cells, and destroy the normal architecture of the lymph node.

There are four histologic categories for Hodgkin's disease. The most common (40% to 60%) histologic subtype of Hodgkin's disease is the **nodular**

177

sclerosing type. The lacunar variant of the Reed-Sternberg cell is present and there is a thickened band of collagen that divides the lymph node into distinct nodules. **Mixed cellularity** occurs in 15% to 30% of cases. In this variant, the Reed-Sternberg cells are abundant and the lymph node is completely effaced, with minimal fibrosis. Less common variants in children are the **lymphocyte-predominant** (5% to 15%) and **lymphocyte-depleted** (<5%) subtypes.

Hodgkin's disease is characterized by progressive enlargement of the lymph nodes with extension to contiguous nodes. Splenic involvement is usually associated with involvement of adjacent lymph nodes. Dissemination may occur hematogenously to involve the bone marrow, liver, lungs, and bone.

Cellular immunodeficiency is present in more than 50% of individuals with Hodgkin's disease and precedes development of the disease. These patients have delayed hypersensitivity on skin testing and increased susceptibility to infection with bacteria, viruses, and fungi. Some recovery of the immune deficiency may occur after successful treatment.

CLINICAL PRESENTATION

More than 90% of children present with painless swelling of one or more groups of superficial lymph nodes, usually in the cervical or supraclavicular area. Unusual sites of adenopathy may be present, such as in the axillary, mediastinal, and retroperitoneal areas. Mediastinal adenopathy may be present in up to 60% of cases and be associated with symptoms such as cough or superior vena cava syndrome. About 30% of children have "B" symptoms, which are systemic symptoms of fever, night sweats, and/or loss of greater than 10% of body weight. The spleen may be enlarged on examination.

DIAGNOSTIC EVALUATION

Following a meticulous history and physical examination, a **biopsy** should be performed on a suspicious lymph node. Typically, adenopathy is first treated with systemic antibiotics for 1 to 2 weeks, and, if the adenopathy persists and is suspicious for malignancy (rubbery, nontender, no site of infection, unusual location, continues to grow), then the next step is referral to a pediatric oncologist and surgeon for evaluation and excisional biopsy. Fine-needle aspirates do not consistently provide adequate material for diagnosis and do not allow for assessment of nodal architecture.

Laboratory studies should include a complete blood count (CBC) with differential; serum chemistries, including liver function tests; and a sedimentation rate (useful for assessment of response to therapy). Other markers for active Hodgkin's disease include elevated levels of serum copper, ferritin, fibrinogen, and alkaline phosphatase. A bone marrow examination is recommended in advanced disease.

Radiographic studies include a chest radiograph to assess for mediastinal adenopathy. For complete staging purposes, a computed tomography

(CT) scan of the neck, chest, abdomen, and pelvis should be done to assess for extent of disease. Additionally, a gallium scan is recommended to assess avidity in the primary tumor site, and ideally should be done prior to excisional biopsy of a single enlarged node. If the tumor is avid, the gallium scan is extremely useful to monitor response to treatment and assess for possible recurrence. Lymphangiogram is recommended by some practitioners but is not available at all centers and is considered to be an invasive procedure.

STAGING

Staging is based on the clinical extent of disease and presence of "B" symptoms:

Stage I: involvement of a single lymph node region or a single extralymphatic site

Stage II: involvement of two or more lymph node regions on the same side of the diaphragm; or localized involvement of extralymphatic organ or site and of one or more lymph node regions on the same side of the diaphragm

Stage III: involvement of lymph node regions on both sides of the diaphragm, which may also be accompanied by localized involvement of extralymphatic organ or site; or by involvement of the spleen; or both

Stage IV: disseminated involvement of one or more extralymphatic organs or tissues with or without lymph node involvement

Patients are designated "A" after the numerical staging in the absence of constitutional symptoms and designated "B" if fever, drenching night sweats, or weight loss exceeding 10% of total body weight is present at diagnosis.

TREATMENT

After surgical biopsy, chemotherapy and/or radiation are the mainstays of therapy. For children in whom growth is not complete, multiagent chemotherapy alone or in combination with involved field radiation is the treatment of choice. Adolescents and adults may receive radiation alone in lower stage disease and multiagent chemotherapy in advanced stages. Drugs active in the treatment of Hodgkin's disease include prednisone, vincristine, procarbazine, cyclophosphamide, vinblastine, Adriamycin, nitrogen mustard, and bleomycin. Treatment usually lasts 4 to 8 months. With current therapy, over 80% of children with Hodgkin's disease may expect to be cured of their disease.

COMPLICATIONS OF THERAPY

Patients receiving therapy for Hodgkin's disease may expect to experience acute and possibly late effects of therapy. Nausea, vomiting, abnormal pulmonary function, and myelosuppression may occur as a result of chemotherapy. Late effects may include impaired fertility, impaired growth, cardiac toxicity, and abnormal pulmonary function dependent on the chemotherapeutic agents used and site of radiation therapy. The risk of second tumors many years following Hodgkin's disease may be related to an underlying immune deficiency and possibly the effects of antitumor therapy.

NON-HODGKIN'S LYMPHOMA

NHLs are about 1.5 times as common as Hodgkin's lymphomas. The incidence in children increases with age, with a steady increase throughout life. The histologic and clinical features of lymphoma differ considerably between children and adults. Childhood lymphomas occur throughout the world, although the relative frequency differs significantly among countries. In equatorial Africa, lymphomas, in particular Burkitt's lymphoma, account for 50% of all childhood malignancies in which EBV is implicated in their development.

Children with congenital or acquired dysfunction of the immune system have a high risk of developing lymphoma. Such conditions include ataxia–telangiectasia, Wiskott-Aldrich, Bloom, and Chédiak-Higashi syndromes, in addition to HIV. Chronic immune suppressive therapy, such as following organ transplant, and chronic treatment with phenytoin are known to increase the risk of developing NHL. EBV is known to be associated with Burkitt's lymphoma and may be causative in Africa. The exact etiology of NHL remains unclear.

There are three major histologic subtypes of NHL in children: large cell, lymphoblastic, and undifferentiated. The large-cell lymphomas tend to be heterogeneous immunologically; most are B-cell derived and some are T-cell derived or arise from the macrophage–histiocyte lineage. Burkitt and non-Burkitt subtypes fall under the category of undifferentiated lymphomas and are virtually all B-cell tumors, distinguished only by the amount of cellular heterogeneity. The most common subtype, lymphoblastic (40%), is predominantly of T-cell origin. All of these subtypes can invade the bone marrow and undergo leukemic transformation.

CLINICAL PRESENTATION

NHLs can arise anywhere in the body, primarily in the lymph nodes, thymus, Waldeyer ring, Peyer patches, and bone marrow. About a third of children have gastrointestinal involvement and present with right lower quadrant pain, nausea, vomiting, and abdominal distention. It is not unusual for NHL to be confused with a surgical abdomen, such as appendicitis. In the United States, Burkitt's lymphomas typically present in the intestine, resulting in an obstruction. Approximately 25% of children have mediastinal involvement with respiratory symptoms, cervical or supraclavicular adenopathy, or superior vena cava syndrome. Children may have very limited disease affecting the tonsils, nasopharynx, or Waldeyer ring, and diagnosis has followed pathologic evaluation after a routine tonsillectomy and adenoidectomy.

DIAGNOSTIC EVALUATION

It is not unusual to begin with a surgical procedure for excision or **biopsy** of a node, or laparotomy in the case of an acute abdominal presentation. Many times the diagnosis is not suspected prior to these procedures. In any event, histologic confirmation is necessary for the diagnosis.

Laboratory studies include a CBC with differential and review of the peripheral smear to assess for possible bone marrow involvement or leukemia, as well as serum chemistries to include liver function studies, blood urea nitrogen, creatinine, lactate dehydrogenase, uric acid, electrolytes, calcium, and phosphorus. Lymphomas, particularly advanced or Burkitt's-type NHL, can present with overt evidence of tumor lysis and/or resultant renal dysfunction. A **bone marrow aspirate** and biopsy should be performed in all patients with confirmed or suspected lymphoma because the child may actually have leukemia (marrow with >25% replacement by lymphoblasts). A **lumbar puncture** to assess the cerebrospinal fluid for involvement of NHL should be done on all children.

Radiographic imaging is dependent on the area of the mass or related symptoms. Initial evaluation should include a chest radiograph and possibly a CT scan of the neck, chest, abdomen, and pelvis.

STAGING

Stage I: a single node or extranodal site, excluding mediastinum and abdomen

Stage II: a single extranodal tumor with regional lymph node involvement; two or more nodal areas on the same side of the diaphragm; resected primary gastrointestinal tumor (usually ileocecal) with or without mesenteric nodes only

Stage III: two or more extranodal sites on both sides of the diaphragm; a primary thoracic tumor; extensive intra-abdominal disease; all paraspinal or epidural tumors

Stage IV: any of the above with dissemination to the central nervous system (CNS) or bone marrow (less than 25% involvement)

TREATMENT

Therapy is based on clinical staging, localized versus disseminated disease, and histologic subtype. In general, children with localized NHL have an excellent prognosis, with a 90% long-term survival. Therapy may begin with surgical resection, as in the case of primary gastrointestinal tumors, though resection is not a necessary part of therapy for treatment of other sites (unless a life-threatening complication is present). These tumors are exquisitely sensitive to chemotherapy, and multidrug regimens, similar to those used for leukemia, are frequently recommended. With the initiation of therapy, the child must be closely monitored for the development of the tumor lysis syndrome and resultant metabolic abnormalities. Some therapeutic regimens begin with a single drug (prednisone) until the time of massive lysis has passed, prior to institution of multidrug therapy. Radiation therapy is not routinely used in the treatment of NHL, but may be useful in treating head and neck tumors. CNS prophylaxis is indicated in advanced stages and in those patients with parameningeal or overt CNS disease at diagnosis. Length of therapy ranges from 6 months to 2 years.

SUGGESTED READING

Diamond CA. Oncology. In: Rudolph AM, Kamei RK (eds), Rudolph's Fundamentals of Pediatrics, 2nd ed. Norwalk, CT: Appleton & Lange, 1998, pp 491–510.

Hudson MM, Donaldson SS. Hodgkin's disease. In: Pizzo PA, Poplack DG (eds), Principles and Practice of Pediatric Oncology, 3rd ed. Philadelphia: Lippincott–Raven, 1997, pp 523–544.

Shad A, Magrath IT. Malignant non-Hodgkin's lymphomas in children. In: Pizzo PA, Poplack DG (eds), Principles and Practice of Pediatric Oncology, 3rd ed. Philadelphia: Lippincott–Raven, 1997, pp 545–588.

WILMS' TUMOR

Wilms' tumor is the second most common retroperitoneal tumor in children, accounting for approximately 6% of childhood malignancies. It is a tumor of the developing kidney and typically occurs in young children between the ages of 1 and 5 years, with equal incidence among boys and girls. Most cases of Wilms' tumor are sporadic, with approximately 1% being familial. Familial cases are more likely bilateral and occur at a younger age.

GENETICS

Congenital anomalies occur in 12% to 15% of cases, the most common anomalies being hemihypertrophy, aniridia, Beckwith-Wiedemann syndrome, and genitourinary tract (GU) anomalies such as cryptorchidism, hypospadias, horseshoe kidney, ureteral duplication, and polycystic kidney. Most children with Wilms' tumor have a normal karyotype; however, a chromosomal deletion in the short arm of chromosome 11 (11p13 deletion) is seen in association with congenital aniridia. The Wilms' tumor 1 (*WT1*) gene encodes a transcription factor important in normal kidney development. Mutations within the *WT1* gene have been identified in two syndromes associated with Wilms' tumor, the WAGR syndrome (Wilms' tumor, aniridia, GU anomalies, and mental retardation), and the Denys-Drash syndrome (Wilms' tumor, nephropathy, and GU anomalies). A second Wilms' tumor gene locus, *WT2*, maps to chromosome 11p15.5. The Beckwith-Wiedemann syndrome also maps to this location. It is likely that other mutations in specific loci may predispose to Wilms' tumor.

CLINICAL PRESENTATION

Abdominal mass is the most common presenting sign and symptom. Associated signs and symptoms include abdominal pain, malaise, hypertension, and microscopic hematuria. Bleeding within the tumor may occur and result in anemia, pallor, and fatigue. Tumor thrombus may extend into the vena cava, causing partial obstruction, hypertension, and distention of abdominal veins. Polycythemia may be seen in Wilms' tumor. Acquired von Willebrand disease (reduced von Willebrand factor, factor VIII coagulant, and ristocetin cofactor levels) has been reported in association with Wilms' tumor and typically resolves with initiation of treatment.

EVALUATION OF SUSPECTED WILMS' TUMOR

- **History:** include family history of malignancies, congenital anomalies
- **Physical examination:** assess for abdominal/flank mass, usually movable; congenital anomalies (hemihypertrophy, GU malformations, aniridia); hypertension; abdominal venous distention; liver enlargement

- **Laboratory studies:** urinalysis with microscopic evaluation, complete blood count (polycythemia, anemia), serum chemistries, coagulation studies
- **Diagnostic imaging studies:**
  1. Abdominal ultrasound to assess intrarenal tumor, possible vena caval involvement, and blood flow
  2. Abdominal computed tomography (CT) with special attention to the opposite kidney, evidence of bilateral involvement, evidence of vessel involvement or extension to the inferior vena cava (IVC), lymph node involvement, liver metastases
  3. Chest radiograph and chest CT to assess for metastases (most common site)
  4. Bone scan indicated if the tumor is a clear cell sarcoma (to assess for metastases)
  5. Magnetic resonance imaging of the brain indicated if the tumor is a rhabdoid or clear cell tumor (to assess for metastases)

- **Chromosome analysis** on the tumor: especially useful in association with congenital anomalies and familial cases
- **Echocardiogram:** useful for detecting tumor extension from the IVC to the right atrium and also indicated if the child is to receive Adriamycin
- **Pathologic diagnosis:**
  1. Surgical removal of the involved kidney and tumor. In some cases, complete removal of the primary tumor may not be possible and biopsy is then indicated (should only be performed by a pediatric surgeon).
  2. Determination of favorable versus unfavorable histology and assessment for anaplasia

STAGING

After the evaluation and surgical staging (includes nephrectomy, assessment of involvement or spread through the renal capsule into the renal pelvis and vessels, and assessment of nodes), the patient is clinically staged. For those patients unable to have a radical nephrectomy because of excessive risk, preoperative chemotherapy or radiation should be given. Eventually the tumor will need to be removed. In these cases, the tumor is considered a stage III tumor locally.

Clinicopathologic staging is as follows:

Stage I: tumor limited to the kidney and completed excised

Stage II: tumor extends through the capsule and into perirenal soft tissue and may infiltrate vessels outside the kidney; completely excised

Stage III: residual nonhematogenous dissemination of tumor confined to the abdomen; tumor may extend beyond surgical margin at resection and may involve lymph node, tumor spill, or peritoneal implants

Stage IV: hematogenous dissemination of tumor to lungs, liver, bone, brain, or distant lymph nodes

Stage V: bilateral renal involvement

Patients with bilateral involvement of tumor (stage V) should have each side independently staged and treatment based on the highest stage.

TREATMENT

The prognosis of Wilms' tumor is very favorable, with more than 85% of children being cured of their disease. Good prognostic factors are low-stage disease, complete surgical resection, favorable histology, and no focal anaplasia. Treatment of Wilms' tumor is based on the most recent recommendations from the National Wilms' Tumor Study (NWTS) group. As the outcome continues to improve, a major goal has been to develop treatment that causes less acute and long-term toxicity. Stage I and II patients with favorable histology and stage I patients with focal anaplasia receive 18 weeks of chemotherapy with two drugs, vincristine and dactinomycin. Patients with stage III and IV disease with favorable histology and those with stage II to IV disease with focal anaplasia receive 24 weeks of chemotherapy with three drugs, vincristine, dactinomycin, and Adriamycin. Additionally, radiation to the local tumor bed and areas of metastasis is recommended. Patients with stage II to IV disease with diffuse anaplasia receive the most aggressive therapy, with 66 weeks of chemotherapy. They receive vincristine, dactinomycin, Adriamycin, and cyclophosphamide in addition to radiation therapy to all sites of disease.

24

TREATMENT

SUGGESTED READING

Diamond CA. Oncology. In: Rudolph AM, Kamei RK (eds), Rudolph's Fundamentals of Pediatrics, 2nd ed. Norwalk, CT: Appleton & Lange, 1998, pp 491–510.

Green DM, Coppes MJ, Breslow NE, et al. Wilms tumor. In: Pizzo PA, Polack DG (eds), Principles and Practice of Pediatric Oncology, 3rd ed. Philadelphia: Lippincott-Raven, 1997, pp 733–760.

NEUROBLASTOMA

25

Neuroblastoma is the most common solid tumor in childhood outside the central nervous system, accounting for 7% of all childhood malignancies. It is the most common tumor in infancy. The peak incidence is 2 years of age. There may be a genetic predisposition for neuroblastoma that has been reported in twins and siblings. The frequency of neuroblastoma is higher in certain conditions, such as the Beckwith-Wiedemann syndrome, nesidioblastosis, neurofibromatosis, Hirschsprung's disease, fetal hydantoin syndrome, fetal alcohol syndrome, familial pheochromocytoma, and heterochromia.

Cytogenetic abnormalities have been detected in neuroblastoma cells, the most common of which is a rearrangement or deletion in the short arm of chromosome 1. Abnormalities are also seen on chromosome 17 in some tumors. The oncogenes n-*myc* and n-*ras* are amplified in neuroblastoma cells. N-*myc* is usually found as a single copy on the short arm of chromosome 2. In many cases of disseminated disease, amplification of the n-*myc* proto-oncogene is found and is a poor prognostic sign.

Neuroblastomas are found with an increased incidence (400-fold over the clinical incidence) in infant autopsies. This suggests that involution or maturation of the tumor occurs spontaneously in most infants. Occasionally, neuroblastoma has been diagnosed on a prenatal ultrasound and removed after birth. The tumor is almost always confined to a single site and has an excellent prognosis.

CLINICAL PRESENTATION

Neuroblastoma originates from primordial neural crest cells that normally give rise to the adrenal medulla and the sympathetic ganglia. It usually presents as a tumor mass along the sympathetic neural pathway. The most common presentation is an abdominal mass with metastases in 70% of cases. The most common site of primary tumors within the abdomen is the adrenal gland, which accounts for 40% of tumors, and the paraspinal ganglion. Tumors can also be found in the neck, thorax, and pelvis. Infants are more likely to have thoracic tumors. Many infants and children present with high-stage disease. Common sites of metastasis are the lymph nodes, bone marrow, bone, liver, and skin.

The signs and symptoms at presentation depend on the site of the tumor, size, and the degree of spread. Abdominal tumors are usually palpable, hard, fixed masses. The liver may be enlarged, leading to respiratory compromise, especially in the infant. There may be evidence of anemia (pallor, weakness, fatigue), a coagulopathy (bruising, bleeding), and bone pain or limping with bone marrow involvement. Thoracic masses are usually picked up in the posterior mediastinum by imaging studies done for other reasons. Cervical masses may be treated as cervical adenopathy related to infection. The presence of Horner's syndrome (contracted pupil, ptosis, enophthalmos, anhidrosis) or heterochromia iridis should prompt an evaluation for cervicothoracic neuroblastoma. Pelvic masses may cause bowel or bladder symptoms. Tumors along the sympathetic ganglia may cause spinal cord compression. Skin lesions tend to be limited to infants and appear as bluish, nontender subcutaneous nodules. Sphenoid or retro-orbital bone involvement may occur and appear clinically as "raccoon eyes" with periorbital hemorrhage. Many children have constitutional symptoms, including weight loss, fever, irritability, lethargy, and anorexia.

An unusual presentation of neuroblastoma is in association with "opsoclonus–myoclonus," also referred to as "dancing eyes–dancing feet." These children have cerebellar and truncal ataxia and rapid eye movements. Developmental delay, language deficits, and behavioral abnormalities may also be present. These children should be carefully evaluated for the presence of an occult neuroblastoma. They tend to have low-stage, highly curable disease, though the impact of cure on the underlying disorder may be minimal, with a high incidence of chronic neurologic deficits. The pathophysiology of this syndrome is not well defined. In addition to treatment of the neuroblastoma, these children may benefit from therapy with dexamethasone and intravenous immune globulin.

DIAGNOSTIC EVALUATION

- **History:** Assess for constitutional symptoms, abdominal pain, bowel or bladder control problems, bleeding, bone pain or limping.
- **Physical examination:** Assess vital signs (fever, hypertension), and evaluate for abdominal mass, spinal cord compression, unusual signs/symptoms associated with neuroblastoma (heterochromia, raccoon eyes, Horner's syndrome), subcutaneous nodules in infants, enlarged liver or lymph nodes, and evidence of anemia or coagulopathy.
- **Laboratory studies:**
  1. Obtain complete blood count with differential, serum chemistries (liver function studies, lactate dehydrogenase), ferritin (may be a tumor marker and elevated in neuroblastoma, though also an acute-phase reactant), and urine for vanillylmandelic acid (VMA) and homovanillic acid (HVA). These urine metabolites are elevated in over 90% of children with neuroblastoma, especially in the higher stages of disease.
  2. Bone marrow aspiration and biopsy (bilateral iliac crests) should be performed to assess for marrow cellularity and investigation of tumor clumps. Special stains are used to differentiate this tumor from other small, round, blue cell tumors of childhood, such as rhabdomyosarcoma, Ewing's sarcoma, lymphoma, and primitive neuroectodermal tumor. Some laboratories offer sophisticated testing for

the presence of neuroblastoma cells at the DNA level; these studies are frequently more useful to assess efficacy of therapy than to aid with diagnosis.

3. A lumbar puncture must be performed in children with a parameningeal or intracranial tumor.

- **Diagnostic imaging studies:** Imaging studies should include a computed tomography scan of the neck, chest, abdomen, and pelvis. Calcifications and hemorrhage are commonly seen, especially in large abdominal masses. The tumors tend to be large and displace adjacent organs; however, the tumor can wrap around major structures, causing obstruction and dysfunction. If there is suspicion of involvement, magnetic resonance imaging of the head or spine should be done. Plain films of all the bones (skeletal survey) and a technetium bone scan are done to assess for bone involvement. Areas of metastasis appear lytic and most often are located in the proximal long bones, orbit, and skull.
- **Biopsy or excision of the tumor:** Localized tumors should be surgically removed. Many tumors are initially unresectable. These tumors should be surgically biopsied, with sampling of local lymph nodes.

The diagnosis may be established by either pathologic diagnosis on tumor tissue *or* positive bone marrow aspirate or biopsy (unequivocal tumor cells by presence of syncytia and immunohistochemistry) *and* increased urine catecholamines or metabolites (VMA and HVA).

STAGING

Stage I: localized tumor confined to the area of origin; complete gross resection, with or without residual disease; negative lymph nodes

Stage IIA: unilateral tumor with incomplete gross resection; negative lymph nodes

Stage IIB: unilateral tumor with complete or incomplete gross resection; positive ipsilateral lymph nodes, negative contralateral lymph nodes

Stage III: tumor infiltrating across midline with or without regional lymph node involvement; or unilateral tumor with contralateral lymph node involvement; or midline tumor with bilateral regional lymph node involvement

Stage IV: tumor disseminated to distant lymph nodes, bone, bone marrow, liver, or other organs (except as defined by stage IVS)

Stage IVS: localized primary tumor as defined for stage I or II with dissemination limited to liver, skin, or bone marrow (typically in a child under 1 year of age)

TREATMENT

Although n-*myc* amplification, unfavorable histology, and DNA ploidy all adversely affect prognosis, treatment is based on the clinical stage and age.

Chemotherapy is the main modality of treatment for all stages of neuroblastoma. Surgery and radiation also have important roles. Infants with stage IVS disease may have spontaneous regression in up to 50% of cases; however, chemotherapy or radiation may be necessary to expedite regression if compression of vital organs occurs. These children need careful observation for progression to stage IV disease and careful assessment of the tumor biology.

Complete surgical resection is an extremely important factor for long-term survival. However, because many children do not have resectable disease at diagnosis, it may serve a diagnostic or palliative function. It is common practice to attempt to shrink the tumor with chemotherapy and then undertake a second-look surgical procedure for an attempt at delayed complete resection. This also provides an opportunity to assess efficacy of the chemotherapy by looking at tumor viability.

Radiation therapy is indicated for primary tumors that cannot be fully resected, sites of metastatic disease (bone), and palliation. The role of intraoperative radiation is being investigated at some centers.

The chemotherapeutic drugs known to be active in neuroblastoma include cyclophosphamide, cisplatin, carboplatin, ifosfamide, doxorubicin, etoposide, and topotecan. Children with advanced disease receive most of these drugs in high doses, using a very aggressive regimen. Autologous bone marrow transplant is offered to children with stage IV disease who have a complete response to initial therapy (surgery and chemotherapy). Many experimental therapies are being investigated, including radioactively labeling drugs that are preferentially taken up by cells producing adrenergic neurotransmitters ([^{131}I]metaiodobenzylguanidine, or MIBG). Retinoic acid, which causes differentiation of neuroblastoma cells, is also being used in advanced disease following chemotherapy or bone marrow transplant.

PROGNOSIS

The most important factors predicting survival are age, clinical stage, n-*myc* amplification, histologic characteristics of the tumor, and clinical response to therapy. Children under 1 year of age without n-*myc* amplification and with a favorable histology have a survival of 95%, irrespective of clinical stage. Children over 1 year of age with advanced disease (stage IV) and n-*myc* amplification have a poor prognosis, with a survival of 25% to 40% following intensive therapy.

SUGGESTED READING

Brodeur GM, Castleberry RP. Neuroblastoma. In: Pizzo PA, Poplack DG (eds), Principles and Practice of Pediatric Oncology, 3rd ed. Philadelphia: Lippincott–Raven, 1997, pp 761–798.

Diamond CA. Oncology. In: Rudolph AM, Kamei RK (eds), Rudolph's Fundamentals of Pediatrics, 2nd ed. Norwalk, CT: Appleton & Lange, 1998, pp 491–510.

GUIDE TO ONCOLOGIC PROCEDURES

All procedures should be performed or instructed by those physicians and nurse practitioners experienced in the techniques. Sterile technique is employed throughout. Have all materials and medications in the room prior to sedation and sterile prep. When sedation is given for a procedure, an additional physician or nurse should be present to monitor the patient, manage IV fluids, and observe the cardiovascular or pulse oximeter monitors. Many programs routinely perform most procedures under a general anesthetic.

26

INTRATHECAL CHEMOTHERAPY

MATERIALS
Lumbar puncture tray
10-ml syringe
22-gauge spinal needle (1½ in. for infants, 2½ in. for older children; longer needles are available)
Betadine and alcohol
Chemotherapy agent
Sterile gloves

All patients must have a platelet count of 30 to 50×10^9/L or greater to have a lumbar puncture. The patient may need to have a platelet transfusion prior to or during the procedure.

PREPARATION
Proper positioning is crucial and requires the assistance of holder(s) to help place the child in a knee-to-chest position to open the vertebral bodies and allow for easier passage of the spinal needle. The patient is placed in the lateral lying or sitting position. The crest of the iliac bone is palpated laterally to assist in finding the L3–4 interspace. Lidocaine-prilocaine (EMLA) cream 2.5 g may be applied topically 1 to 2 hours prior to the procedure for local anesthesia, and is wiped off prior to the sterile preparation. The area is prepped with three povidone-iodine (Betadine) scrubs and alcohol wipes, then draped sterilely. An assistant transfers the chemotherapy agent by attaching a needle to the chemotherapy syringe and transferring the contents sterilely into a new syringe held by the person performing the procedure. **Ensure that the label is rechecked for drug, dose, mode of infusion, and patient identification.**

TECHNIQUE

Lidocaine 1% may be given (with sodium bicarbonate to cut the sting of the lidocaine in a dilution of 4:1 lidocaine to bicarbonate) SQ at the site prior to puncture with the spinal needle. It may not be indicated in the small child because of prominence of landmarks, anxiety, and anticipated ease of procedure.

The spinal needle is then inserted with a stylet until a "give" or "pop" is felt and then the stylet is removed. In children who have experienced numerous lumbar punctures, there may be no give or the needle may encounter tough fibrous tissue on the way in. The experienced assistant will help with the determination of how far to insert the needle. Observe for flow of cerebrospinal fluid (CSF); the CSF should be clear with a good, steady flow. If the flow is very slow, rotate the spinal needle 45 degrees and observe. The quantity of CSF removed should closely approximate the quantity of chemotherapy agent to be given (standard is 4 to 6 ml). Collect the fluid in two tubes.

The syringe with the chemotherapy agent is then securely attached to the hub of the spinal needle, without advancing or pulling back on the needle. The syringe will need to be firmly screwed on. Gently press the syringe plunger and administer the chemotherapy agent over 2 to 4 minutes. It should flow easily and without resistance. Chemotherapy should not be administered when any of the following situations exist: the spinal fluid is bloody, indicating puncture of a vessel with possible leakage of chemotherapy agent; the child is moving too much to make it a safe procedure; the chemotherapy agent does not advance easily and, when checked again, the flow of CSF has stopped or greatly diminished; the chemotherapy agent or dose is incorrect; or the child experiences pain with injection.

After administration of chemotherapy, the syringe is detached, the stylet replaced, and the needle with stylet removed. The area is cleansed and dried and a spot bandage applied.

The patient is then instructed to stay in a lying position (preferably mild Trendelenburg) for 1 hour. If still moderately sedated, the child should return to his/her room with a pulse oximeter, cardiovascular monitor, and frequent nursing checks and vital signs.

The CSF obtained is immediately taken to the laboratory and cytocentrifuged. A sample is taken for a cell count and cytology. Protein and glucose levels are only determined on initial taps and CSF from patients with a history of abnormalities. Cultures are only done if the patient is febrile or culture is clinically indicated.

DOCUMENTATION

Document in the patient's chart the details of the procedure (including sedation), the chemotherapy agent administered, the specimen collected, and patient tolerance of the procedure.

INTRA-OMMAYA RESERVOIR TAP AND INJECTION OF CHEMOTHERAPY

MATERIALS

Lumbar puncture tray
25-gauge butterfly needle
2 syringes—5 and 3 ml
Mask
Razor
Antibacterial soap and 4×4 sterile gauze
Chemotherapy agent
Sterile gloves

PREPARATION

The patient is placed in a supine or sitting position. If needed, the reservoir area is shaved. Wearing a mask and sterile gloves, clean the reservoir site with sterile gauze and an antibacterial soap in a circular fashion, three times. Change gloves, then continue with a routine sterile prep with three Betadine scrubs and alcohol wipes.

Sterilely transfer (as for intrathecal chemotherapy above) the chemotherapy agent (after checking for drug, patient, and dose) into a 5-ml syringe and the normal saline flush into a 3-ml syringe. Apply sterile drapes, if used.

TECHNIQUE

Topical EMLA cream 2.5 g may have been applied earlier for topical anesthesia; otherwise no sedation or local anesthesia is usually necessary. Puncture the reservoir site with a 25-gauge butterfly needle. The CSF is allowed to drip (or is slowly withdrawn) from the butterfly needle into a sterile tube. The total volume collected should approximate the total volume to be given (chemotherapy agent plus normal saline flush). The chemotherapy agent is injected over 2 to 3 minutes. Do not give the drug if the CSF is blood tinged.

The needle is removed and firm pressure is applied to the site for several minutes. A spot bandage is applied.

DOCUMENTATION

Document in the patient's chart the details of the procedure, the chemotherapy agent administered, the specimen collected, and the patient's status after the procedure.

BONE MARROW ASPIRATE AND BIOPSY

MATERIALS

Biopsy tray with Betadine, alcohol, gauze, 20-ml syringes (two to four depending on indication), 16-gauge aspirate needle, 11-gauge 4 in. or 13-gauge 3½ in. Jamshidi biopsy needle (or similar)

26

BONE MARROW ASPIRATE AND BIOPSY

EDTA to coat syringes (anticoagulant)
Technician present

Bone marrow aspirates and biopsies are usually done on the largest accessible bones in the body, the posterior iliac crests. They may be done in unusual locations for special situations (infants, children on ventilators, etc.).

PREPARATION
The patient is placed in the prone position with a small lift under the hip to accentuate the posterior iliac crests.

TECHNIQUE
EMLA cream 2.5 g is applied topically 1 to 2 hours before the procedure to the spine of the posterior iliac crest (if the patient will be awake). The patient is appropriately sedated if necessary. Topical anesthesia is further achieved with lidocaine 1% (and sodium bicarbonate 4:1 ratio as above) injected locally (2 to 3 ml depending on size of the child) to the depth of the periosteum.

A 16-gauge Monoject aspirate (or similar) needle is used. It is placed into the skin at an angle and then, once through the skin, placed perpendicular to the iliac crest. With gradual pressure, insert the needle with the stylet in place into the iliac crest. Once through the cortex, the needle will "give" as it enters the marrow space and a crunching sound or feeling may be appreciated. The stylet is removed, and the needle should remain firmly in place. The 20-ml syringe (coated with ethylenediaminetetra-acetic acid [EDTA] to avoid clotting) is firmly attached to the hub of the needle. Holding onto both the needle and syringe, pressure is applied to draw up marrow into the syringe. The patient may experience a sensation down the legs at the time of aspiration. Aspirate approximately 1 to 2 ml of marrow, then detach the syringe carefully and hand immediately to the technician for quick visual inspection for marrow tissue (fat, spicules). Once this has been confirmed, obtain additional marrow as needed, then reinsert the stylet and remove the needle. Apply pressure for several minutes and then a pressure bandage.

For biopsy, the same principles of sterile preparation and anesthesia apply. The biopsy needle is inserted with the trocar in the same manner as above, though, once anchored into the cortex, the trocar is removed. The needle is then inserted through the depth of the cortex and into the marrow 5 to 10 mm (depending on size of the child). The needle is then rocked at all angles to break off the core biopsy sample at the base and the needle is removed. The accompanying stylet (no sharp edge) is inserted at the sharp end of the needle and the core tissue biopsy pushed out gently onto sterile gauze. It is then examined for the presence of adequate marrow tissue and given to the technician to place in fixative. Again, pressure is applied for several minutes, followed with a pressure bandage.

DOCUMENTATION
Document in the patient's chart the details of the procedure (including sedation) and specimens collected, in addition to the patient's clinical status during and after the procedure.

ADMINISTRATION OF PERIPHERAL CHEMOTHERAPY (IN A CHILD WITHOUT A CENTRAL VENOUS CATHETER)

MATERIALS
Chemotherapy agent (premixed by pharmacy in syringe)
Stopcock
25-gauge butterfly needle
Alcohol wipes
Gauze (2×2)
Tourniquet
10-ml saline flush
Band-Aid
Gloves (optional)

Review the patient's chemotherapy regimen to determine what medication(s) need(s) to be administered and approve dose(s). Verify the labels on the syringe(s) of the drug(s) against the patient's chart and orders to ensure accuracy. Check to make sure that laboratory criteria have been met (e.g., absolute neutrophil count, liver functions) as determined by the chemotherapy regimen.

PREPARATION
Prepare the child for the procedure. The child may either sit or lie down during the procedure. Explain the procedure, taking into account the child's age, developmental status, and prior experience. Elicit the child's help by encouraging him/her to hold as still as possible. Let him/her know it is okay to cry. Explain each step as you go.

TECHNIQUE
Assemble equipment: attach the butterfly needle to the stopcock, attach the chemotherapy syringe to the *right* side of the stopcock, attach the normal saline (NS) syringe to the remaining junction of the stopcock, and flush the stopcock and butterfly needle with NS.

Wash hands. Select an appropriate vein, preferably on the dorsum of the hand or foot. Avoid the antecubital fossae or joint spaces because of the possibility of deep extravasation of the chemotherapy agent. EMLA cream may be applied 1 hour prior to the procedure, but may cause vasoconstriction of the vein.

Apply the tourniquet. Clean the insertion area with alcohol. Let the area air dry or wipe dry with clean gauze. Insert the butterfly needle with the bevel pointed UP. Advance the needle until blood returns. When blood re-

26

ADMINISTRATION OF PERIPHERAL CHEMOTHERAPY

turns, remove the tourniquet, connect the stopcock, and flush with 2 to 3 ml of NS. If no sign of infiltration occurs (e.g., pain, swelling) and blood return continues, administer the chemotherapy agent slowly via IV push, checking intermittently every 10 to 15 seconds for blood return or swelling. When chemotherapy administration is completed, flush with remaining NS. Remove the butterfly needle and apply pressure for 1 to 2 minutes with clean gauze. Apply Band-Aid.

If infiltration has occurred, see Chapter 27.

DOCUMENTATION

Document in the patient's chart the indication for and details of the procedure, medication, dosage, site, and any complications.

TREATMENT OF CHEMOTHERAPY EXTRAVASATIONS

Extravasation is the leakage of an intravenous drug into the surrounding tissues. Reactions of an extravasation of a vesicant chemotherapy agent can range from mild pain and erythema to tissue necrosis, ulceration, and damage to tendons and nerves.

27

The incidence of vesicant extravasation injury ranges from 0.5% to 6%. Treatment of an extravasation is determined by the particular chemotherapy agent involved (Table 27–1), but remains controversial because the majority of studies have been done on animal models.

The anthracyclines (daunomycin and doxorubicin) and mechlorethamine (nitrogen mustard) bind to DNA. As the cells die, the drug is released and enters undamaged cells. This increases the area of damage and slows healing. Injuries from doxorubicin may continue for weeks.

The vinca alkaloids (vinblastine, vincristine, vindesine) do not bind DNA. The area of damage is less, resembles a chemical burn, and heals more quickly.

Factors that place children at risk for extravasation include poor vein selection, multiple venous punctures to establish a patent IV, obesity, dehy-

TABLE 27–1

EXTRAVASATION TREATMENT

AGENT EXTRAVASATED	COLD/WARM PACK	ANTIDOTE
Anthracyclines Daunomycin Doxorubicin	Cold pack. Apply for 15 minutes 4–6 times/day × 48 hours. Elevate.	None
Dactinomycin	Cold pack. Apply for 15 minutes 4–6 times/day × 48 hours. Elevate. **NOTE:** Heat may increase damage.	None
Mechlorethamine	Cold pack. Apply for 15 minutes 4–6 times/day × 48 hours. Elevate.	Sodium thiosulfate: 1:6 M solution. Mix 4 ml of 10% solution with 6 ml sterile water. Inject 2 ml SQ for each 1 mg of mechlorethamine.
Vinca alkaloids Vinblastine Vincristine Vindesine	Warm packs. Apply for 15 minutes 4–6 times/ day × 48 hours. Elevate.	Hyaluronidase: 150 units in 1 ml normal saline. Give 0.2 ml SQ or intra-dermally into the site or leading edge × 5.

dration, inability to report pain at the injection site, and inexperience of the chemotherapy administrator.

SUGGESTED READING

Fischer DS, Tish Knobf MK, Durivage HJ. The Cancer Chemotherapy Handbook, 4th ed. St. Louis: Mosby, 1993, pp 464–468.

Fishman M, Mrozek-Orlowski M (eds). Cancer Chemotherapy Guidelines and Recommendations for Practice, 2nd ed. Pittsburgh: Oncology Nursing Press, 1999, pp 32–41.

Mullin S, Beckwith MC, Tyler LS. Prevention and management of antineoplastic extravasation injury. Hosp Pharmacy 35:57–74, 2000.

Murphy JS, Willoughby MLN. The management of drug extravasation. In: Ablin AR (ed), Supportive Care of Children with Cancer, 2nd ed. Baltimore: The Johns Hopkins University Press, 1997, pp 112–117.

Formulary Index

Generic Name	Trade Name
Acyclovir	Zovirax
Allopurinol	Zyloprim
Alteplase (tissue plasminogen activator [t-PA])	Activase
Amifostine	Ethyol
Aminocaproic acid	Amicar
Amphotericin B	Fungizone
Amphotericin B cholesteryl sulfate	Amphotec
Amphotericin B lipid complex	Abelcet
Amphotericin B, liposomal	AmBisome
Asparaginase (L-asparaginase)	Elspar
Bleomycin sulfate	Blenoxane
Busulfan	Myleran
Carboplatin	Paraplatin
Carmustine (BCNU)	BiCNU
Cisplatin	Platinol
Cyclophosphamide	Cytoxan
Cyclosporine	Sandimmune
Cytarabine hydrochloride (Ara-C)	Cytostar
Dacarbazine	DTIC
Dactinomycin (actinomycin D)	Cosmegan
Daunorubicin hydrochloride	Cerubidine
Deferoxamine mesylate	Desferal
Desmopressin acetate	DDAVP, Stimate
Dexamethasone	Decadron
Dimercaprol	BAL
Diphenhydramine	Benadryl
Doxorubicin hydrochloride	Adriamycin
Dronabinol	Marinol
Edetate calcium disodium (EDTA)	Calcium Disodium Versenate
Enoxaparin	Lovenox
Epoetin alfa (erythropoietin)	Epogen, Procrit
Etoposide (VP-16)	VePesid
Eutectic mixture of lidocaine and prilocaine	EMLA
Ferrous gluconate	Fergon
Ferrous sulfate	Feosol, Fer-In-Sol
Filgrastim (G-CSF)	Neupogen

Generic Name	Trade Name
Fluconazole	Diflucan
Folic acid (folate)	Folvite
Granisetron	Kytril
Heparin sodium	Lipo-Hepin, Hep-Lock
Hyaluronidase	Wydase
Hydrocortisone	Hydrocortone, Solu-Cortef, Cortef
Hydromorphone hydrochloride	Dilaudid
Hydroxyurea	Hydrea
Idarubicin	Idamycin
Ifosfamide	Ifex
Immune globulin (IV)	Gamimune N, Gammagard, Sandoglobulin, Venoglobulin, Polygam
Iron dextran complex	Imferon
Iron complex (polysaccharide)	Niferex
Ketorolac tromethamine	Toradol
Leucovorin calcium	Wellcovorin
Lomustine (CCNU)	CeeNU
Meperidine hydrochloride	Demerol
Mercaptopurine (6-MP)	Purinethol
Mesna	Mesnex
Methadone hydrochloride	Dolophine
Methotrexate	Mexate
Methylprednisolone	Depo-Medrol, Solu-Medrol
Metoclopramide	Reglan
Morphine sulfate	Astramorph/PF, Duramorph, MS Contin
Naloxone	Narcan
Ondansetron	Zofran
Pegaspargase (PEG-L-asparaginase)	Oncaspar
Pentamidine isethionate	Pentam 300, NebuPent
Prednisone	Deltasone, Meticorten, Orasone
Procarbazine hydrochloride	Matulane
Rh_o (D) immune globulin (IV)	WinRho SD
Sargramostim (GM-CSF)	Leukine, Prokine
Succimer	Chemet (2,3-dimercaptosuccinic acid; DMSA)
Sulfamethoxazole and Trimethoprim (SMX-TMP)	Bactrim, Bactrim DS, Septra, Septra DS
Thioguanine (6-TG)	
Thiotepa	Thioplex
Thrombin, topical	
Tranexamic acid	Cyklokapron
Urate oxidase	Rasburicase

Generic Name	Trade Name
Urokinase	Abbokinase, Abbokinase Open-Cath
Vinblastine sulfate	Velban
Vincristine sulfate	Oncovin
Vitamin K_1/phytonadione	AquaMEPHYTON, Mephyton
Warfarin sodium	Coumadin

FORMULARY

Formulary

Sample entry:

Generic name
Trade and other names
Drug category
How supplied
Pregnancy category (see explanation below)
Indications
Dosage
Contraindications, including adverse events, monitoring, and dose
  modification

Pregnancy categories:

A: Adequate studies in pregnant women have not demonstrated a risk to
  the fetus in the first trimester of pregnancy and there is no evidence of
  risk in later trimesters.
B: Animal studies have not demonstrated a risk to the fetus, but there are
  no adequate studies in pregnant women; or animal studies have shown
  an adverse effect, but adequate studies in pregnant women have not
  demonstrated a risk to the fetus during the first trimester of pregnancy,
  and there is no evidence of risk in later trimesters.
C: Animal studies have shown an adverse effect on the fetus, but there are
  no adequate studies in humans; or there are no animal reproduction
  studies and no adequate studies in humans.
D: There is evidence of human fetal risk, but the potential benefits from the
  use of the drug in pregnant women may be acceptable despite its potential risk.
X: Studies in animals or humans demonstrate fetal abnormalities or adverse reaction; reports indicate evidence of fetal risk. The risk of use in
  a pregnant woman clearly outweighs any possible benefit.

ACYCLOVIR
Zovirax
Antiviral
Capsules: 200 mg
Suspension: 200 mg/5 ml
Injection: 500-mg vial
Pregnancy category C

Indications:
Treatment of initial and prophylaxis for recurrent mucosal and cutaneous herpes simplex virus (HSV-1 and HSV-2) infections, herpes simplex encephalitis, herpes zoster infections, and varicella zoster infections.

Dosage:
Children and neonates:
Mucocutaneous HSV: 750 mg/m^2/day IV divided q8h or 15 to 25 mg/kg/day IV divided q8h for 5 to 10 days
HSV encephalitis: 1500 mg/m^2/day IV divided q8h or 30 to 50 mg/kg/day IV divided q8h for 10 days

Neonatal HSV: 1500 mg/m^2/day IV divided q8h or 30 to 50 mg/kg/day IV divided q8h for 10 to 14 days
Varicella zoster: 1500 mg/m^2/day IV divided q8h or 30 to 50 mg/kg/day IV divided q8h for 5 to 10 days

Contraindications:
Adjust dose in renal impairment. Adequate hydration and slow IV (1 hour) administration are essential to prevent crystallization in the renal tubules. Oral absorption is unpredictable (15% to 30%). Use ideal body weight for obese patients when calculating dosage.

ALLOPURINOL
Zyloprim
Genitourinary, antigout agent
Tablets: 100 and 300 mg
Injection: 500 mg/ml
Pregnancy category C

Indications:
Treatment of secondary hyperuricemia, which may occur as a result of tumor lysis syndrome; prevention of recurrent calcium oxalate calculi; prevention of gouty arthritis and nephropathy.

Dosage:
Under 10 years of age: 10 mg/kg/day PO divided q8h or 300 mg/m^2/day divided q8h

10 years of age to adult:
PO: 100 to 200 mg/day divided in 2 to 3 doses; 600 to 800 mg/day for the prevention of acute uric acid nephropathy (800 mg/day maximum dose)

IV (investigational): 300 to 500 mg/m^2/day divided q8h, not to exceed 800 mg/day

Contraindications:
Reduce dosage in renal impairment; discontinue with rash (may be exacerbated with ampicillin or amoxicillin). Risk of hypersensitivity may be increased in patients receiving thiazides/angiotensin-converting enzyme inhibitors. May cause rash, neuritis, gastrointestinal disturbance, hepatotoxicity, bone marrow suppression, and drowsiness.

ALTEPLASE (Tissue plasminogen activator [t-pa])

Activase
Thrombolytic
Powder for injection: 20 mg (11.6 million units)/20 ml; 50 mg (29 million units)/50 ml
Pregnancy category C

Indications:

Treatment of recent severe or massive deep vein (DVT) or arterial thrombosis, pulmonary embolus, or occluded venous catheters.

Dosage:

Pulmonary embolus, DVT, central venous thrombosis, superior vena cava syndrome: 0.1 mg/kg/hour IV for 6 hours, re-evaluate patient and assess fibrinogen. If no response, sequentially increase doses by 0.05 to 0.1 mg/kg/hour for 6 hours (maximum dose 0.5 mg/kg/hour; maximum daily dose 100 mg). In the case of a pulmonary embolus, a bolus of 0.25 to 0.5 mg/kg may be administered over 10 to 20 minutes, followed by an infusion as above. Maximum duration of therapy is 72 hours or based on the patient's clinical course. Preferable to infuse thrombolytic agent close to site of thrombus.
Occluded central venous catheters (CVCs):
  Under 3 months of age: 0.25 mg IV (0.5 ml)

Over 3 months of age: 0.5 mg IV (1 ml)
Instill a dose in each lumen of a CVC, allow to dwell for 30 minutes. If unsuccessful, repeat dose. If the CVC remains obstructed, begin 6-hour infusion with 0.01 mg/kg/hour. Dose may be increased sequentially to 0.03 to 0.05 mg/kg/hour (maximum dose 1 mg/hour). Maximum length of therapy is 24 hours, depending on the patient's clinical course.
Purpura fulminans: 0.5 mg/kg IV infusion over 1 hour, followed by 0.25 mg/kg hour over 3 hours (total dose 1.25 mg/kg over 4 hours)

Contraindications:

Avoid central venous puncture and noncompressible arterial sticks during infusions. Avoid use in excessive hypertension, recent (within 1 month) cerebral vascular accident, gastrointestinal bleeding, trauma, surgery, bleeding diathesis, or suspicion of a subarachnoid hemorrhage.

AMIFOSTINE
Ethyol
Antidote/deterrent
Injection: 500-mg vial
Pregnancy category C

Indications:
An investigational cryoprotective drug that may reduce the toxicity of radiation and alkylating agents such as cisplatin and cyclophosphamide.

Dosage:
Refer to individual protocol. Usual dosage is 740 to 910 mg/m^2 IV over 15 to 30 minutes prior to a dose of cisplatin or alkylating agent.

Contraindications:
Avoid in hypotension or dehydration. Can cause severe nausea and vomiting and usually requires antiemetic premedication.

AMINOCAPROIC ACID
Amicar
Antihemorrhagic
Tablet: 500 mg
Syrup: 1.25 gm/5 ml (= 250 mg/ml)
Injection: 250 mg/ml (20 ml)
Pregnancy category C

Indications:
Treatment of excessive bleeding resulting from excessive activity of the fibrinolytic system. Typically used to treat mucosal-type bleeding in patients with bleeding diatheses (von Willebrand disease, hemophilia).

Dosage:
PO/IV: 100 to 200 mg/kg as an initial dose (maximum 10 g), followed by 50 to 100 mg/kg/dose (maximum 5 g) every 6 hours. Treat until symptoms resolve (1 to 14 days).
Continuous IV infusion: Loading dose of 100 mg/kg, then 10 to 33 mg/kg/hour in 5% dextrose in water (maximum 1.25 g/hour).

Contraindications:
May accumulate in patients with decreased renal function. Avoid in patients with hematuria. Increased risk of thrombosis with oral contraceptives, estrogens, and factor IX.

AMPHOTERICIN B

Fungizone
Antifungal
Injection: 50-mg vial
Pregnancy category B

Indications:

Treatment of severe systemic infections and meningitis caused by susceptible fungi such as *Candida* species, *Histoplasma capsulatum, Cryptococcus neoformans, Aspergillus* species, *Blastomyces dermatitidis, Torulopsis glabrata*, and *Coccidioides immitis*. Also used empirically to treat suspected invasive fungal disease in immune compromised hosts with prolonged fever.

Dosage:

Test dose of 0.1 mg/kg to a maximum of 1 mg IV over 20 to 60 minutes; an alternative is to initiate therapy with 0.25 mg/kg IV over 2 to 4 hours with frequent observation of the patient and vital signs. If the infusion is well tolerated after a test dose, a therapeutic dose of 0.4 mg/kg can be given on the same day. If the higher dose is well tolerated, 0.25 mg/kg may be given again, usually 12 hours later.

The daily dose is increased by 0.25 mg/kg until the desired daily dose is reached. In critically ill patients, rapid escalation of dosing may be needed.

Daily empiric dose is 0.6 mg/kg/day and daily therapeutic dose for confirmed invasive fungal infection is 0.6 to 1 mg/kg/day. Daily infusion is over 2 to 6 hours, depending on infusion tolerability. Saline boluses pre- and postinfusion often help prevent excessive hypokalemia. Premedication is frequently needed with acetaminophen or diphenhydramine, and, if the patient experiences rigors, meperidine hydrochloride may be given. Once therapy has been established, alternate-day dosing may be administered at a dose of 1 to 1.5 mg/kg/day.

Contraindications:

Because of the nephrotoxic potential of this drug, avoidance of other nephrotoxic medications is advised, if possible. Monitor daily electrolytes, renal function studies, and urine output. Common metabolic abnormalities include hypokalemia, hypomagnesemia, and hypocalcemia. Other problems that may occur are thrombocytopenia, hyperglycemia, diarrhea, dyspnea, back pain, and increases in transaminases and bilirubin. Common infusion-related toxicities are fever, chills, rigors, nausea, vomiting, hypotension, and headache. Imidazole derivatives (e.g., miconazole, fluconazole, ketoconazole) may antagonize the effect and induce fungal resistance to amphotericin.

AMPHOTERICIN B CHOLESTERYL SULFATE
Amphotec
Antifungal
Injection: 50- and 100-mg vial
Pregnancy category B

Indications:
Treatment of invasive fungal disease in patients who are refractory to or intolerant of conventional amphotericin B.

Dosage:
Start at 3 to 4 mg/kg/day and increase to 6 mg/kg/day if necessary. A test dose of 10 ml of the diluted solution over 15 to 30 minutes is recommended. Give first dose at 1 mg/kg/hour; if well tolerated, the infusion time can be gradually decreased to 2 hours.

Contraindications:
See Amphotericin B.

AMPHOTERICIN B LIPID COMPLEX
Abelcet
Antifungal
Injection: 100 mg/20 ml
Pregnancy category B

Indications:
Treatment of aspergillosis or invasive fungal infection in patients who are refractory to or intolerant of conventional amphotericin B therapy. Patients with acute or pre-existing renal toxicity (serum creatinine level double that of baseline) should be considered to receive this product in lieu of conventional amphotericin B. May be useful in the treatment of hepatosplenic candidiasis and cryptococcal meningitis.

Dosage:
Usual dose is 2.5 to 5 mg/kg IV once daily over 2 hours. Rate should not exceed 2.5 mg/kg/hour.

Contraindications:
See Amphotericin B.

AMPHOTERICIN B, LIPOSOMAL
AmBisome
Antifungal
Injection: 50-mg vial
Pregnancy category B

Indications:
Treatment of invasive fungal infection in patients intolerant of or refractory to conventional amphotericin B.

Dosage:
Usual dose is 3 to 5 mg/kg/day IV over 2 hours. Infusion may be shortened to 1 hour if well tolerated.

Contraindications:
See Amphotericin B.

ASPARAGINASE (L-Asparaginase)
Elspar
Antineoplastic
Injection: 10,000-unit vial (*Escherichia coli*)
            10,000-unit vial (*Erwinia*)
Pregnancy category C

Indications:
Treatment of acute lymphoblastic leukemia (ALL), acute myelogenous leukemia, and lymphoma.

Dosage:
Refer to individual protocol. Usual dose for induction for ALL is 6000 units/m^2 IM three times a week for 9 doses. High-dose protocols may give 15,000 to 20,000 U/m^2. Maximum 2-ml volume per injection site. May need multiple injections for a large dose.

Patients should be observed in a clinic or hospital setting for at least 1 hour after administration to assess for allergic reaction.

Contraindications:
Pancreatitis; prior significant hemorrhagic event associated with asparaginase. Hypersensitivity to *E. coli* asparaginase may necessitate switch to the investigational *Erwinia* form of asparaginase. Asparaginase may cause hyperglycemia, hyperuricemia, hyperammonemia, hypofibrinogenemia, thrombosis, hemorrhage, anaphylaxis, and hemorrhagic cystitis.

BLEOMYCIN SULFATE
Blenoxane
Antineoplastic antibiotic
Injection: 15-unit vial (1 unit = 1 mg)
Pregnancy category D

Indications:
Treatment of Hodgkin's disease, sarcomas, and germ cell tumors.

Dosage:
Refer to individual protocol. Usual dose is 10 to 20 U/m² IV one to two times per week and 15 to 20 U/m²/day for 4 to 5 days. Test dose recommended for lymphoma patients (1 to 2 units for the first 2 doses; if well tolerated, give remainder of dose 1 hour later). Administer over at least 10 minutes, not to exceed 1 U/minute. May be given as continuous IV infusion in some protocols.

Contraindications:
Hypersensitivity to bleomycin. Dose may need to be modified for renal or pulmonary toxicity. Monitor renal function studies and pulmonary function, including forced expiratory volume in 1 minute, forced vital capacity, and carbon monoxide diffusion in lungs. May decrease phenytoin concentration. Cisplatin decreases clearance of bleomycin.

BUSULFAN
Myleran
Antineoplastic
Tablet: 2 mg
Pregnancy category D

Indications:
Treatment of chronic myelogenous leukemia (CML) and as a part of a marrow-ablative conditioning regimen prior to bone marrow transplant.

Dosage:
Refer to individual protocol.
For CML induction: 0.06 to 0.12 mg/kg once daily or 1.8 to 4.6 mg/m²/day
For marrow-ablative conditioning regimen: 1 mg/kg/dose q6h for 16 doses.

Contraindications:
Hypersensitivity to busulfan; should not be used in pregnancy or nursing. May cause severe myelosuppression. Use with caution with other myelosuppressive drugs or radiation. May cause hemorrhagic cystitis. Use with thioguanine may increase hepatic toxicity.

CARBOPLATIN
Paraplatin
Antineoplastic
Injection: 50-, 150-, and 450-mg vials
Pregnancy category D

Indications:
Treatment of pediatric brain tumors, neuroblastoma, testicular tumors, relapsed leukemia or solid tumors.

Dosage:
Refer to individual protocol.
Solid tumors: dose is typically 320 to 560 mg/m^2 every 3 to 4 weeks
Brain tumor protocols: 175 mg/m^2/week for 4 weeks, then 2 weeks off
  Dose adjusted based on suppression of neutrophil and platelet counts or renal toxicity.

Contraindications:
Hypersensitivity to carboplatin, cisplatin, or other platinum-containing compounds. Severe marrow suppression or vomiting may occur. Reduce dose in impaired renal function (creatinine clearance <60 ml/minute). Aminoglycosides may increase ototoxicity and nephrotoxicity; nephrotoxic drugs may increase renal toxicity of carboplatin.

CARMUSTINE (BCNU)
BiCNU
Alkylating agent
Injection: 100-mg vial
Pregnancy category D

Indications:
Palliative treatment of brain tumors and treatment of Hodgkin's and non-Hodgkin's lymphomas.

Dosage:
Refer to individual protocol. Typical dose may be 100 to 250 mg/m^2/dose IV every 4 to 6 weeks.

Contraindications:
Hypersensitivity to carmustine. Severe marrow suppression may necessitate change in dosing for subsequent cycles. Pulmonary toxicity in patients receiving more than a 1400 mg/m^2 cumulative dose. Cimetidine potentiates myelosuppressive effects.

CISPLATIN
Platinol
Antineoplastic
Injection: 50-mg vials
Pregnancy category D

Indications:
Treatment of sarcomas, osteosarcoma, Hodgkin's and non-Hodgkin's lymphomas, brain tumors, germ cell tumors, and neuroblastoma.

Dosage:
Refer to individual protocol.
Infants: 1.3 to 3.5 mg/kg/day
Children:
Neuroblastoma: 15 to 30 mg/m^2 for 4 days
Rhabdomyosarcoma: 90 to 100 mg/m^2 as a single dose
Osteosarcoma: 120 mg/m^2 or 3 mg/kg as a single dose
Germ cell tumor: 20 to 40 mg/m^2/day for 5 days

Medulloblastoma: 100 mg/m^2 as a single dose

The rate of intravenous infusion is dose dependent and ranges from a 15- to 20-minute infusion to a 6- to 8-hour infusion or a 24-hour infusion.

Contraindications:
Hypersensitivity to cisplatin or platinum-containing compounds; pre-existing renal impairment; hearing impairment; myelosuppression. Increased risk of nephrotoxicity when given with other nephrotoxic drugs (aminoglycosides, amphotericin B); reduces renal elimination of methotrexate. Increased risk of ototoxicity with loop diuretics and aminoglycosides.

CYCLOPHOSPHAMIDE
Cytoxan
Alkylating agent
Tablets: 25 and 50 mg
Injection: 100 and 500 mg; 1-g vials
Pregnancy category C

Indications:
Treatment of Hodgkin's disease, lymphomas, leukemias, and neuroblastoma; preconditioning therapy for bone marrow transplant; treatment of nephrotic syndrome, lupus erythematosus, and rheumatic diseases.

Dosage:
Refer to individual protocol.
Low-dose regimens: 60 to 600 mg/m²/
    dose IV
High-dose regimens: 15 to 50 mg/kg/
    dose or 1200 to 4000 mg/m²/dose

May be given 1 to 5 mg/kg/day orally for treatment of nephrotic syndrome and some malignancies.

Contraindications:
Hypersensitivity to cyclophosphamide; dose may need to be adjusted for myelosuppression or impaired renal function. High-dose therapy may need to be given with mesna for uroprotection. Allopurinol may increase the myelotoxicity of cyclophosphamide by inhibiting its metabolism.

CYCLOSPORINE

Sandimmune
Immune suppressant
Capsules: 25, 50, and 100 mg
Solution: 100 mg/ml
Injection: 50 mg/ml
Pregnancy category C

Indications:
Used with corticosteroids to prolong organ and patient survival in kidney, liver, heart, and bone marrow transplants; treatment of aplastic anemia.

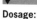

Dosage:
Oral:
Initial: 14 to 18 mg/kg/dose daily, beginning 4 to 12 hours prior to organ transplantation
Maintenance: 10 to 25 mg/kg/day as a single dose, decrease by 5% per week to 5 to 10 mg/kg/day
IV:
Initial: 1 to 6 mg/kg/day every 12 to 24 hours. Adjust dose according to whole-blood high-performance liquid chromatography trough concentrations to keep between 100 and 200 ng/ml.

Maintenance: 5 to 9 mg/kg/day every 12 to 24 hours

Contraindications:
Hypersensitivity to cyclosporine (castor oil is an ingredient in the preparation). Requires close monitoring of renal and hepatic function. Drug interactions include ketoconazole, itraconazole, fluconazole, erythromycin, and methylprednisolone, which increase the cyclosporine concentration by inhibiting hepatic metabolism. Acyclovir, aminoglycosides, trimethoprim–sulfamethoxazole, melphalan, and amphotericin B may increase nephrotoxicity. Cimetidine may increase cyclosporine concentration. Refer to *Physicians' Desk Reference* for extensive drug interaction information.

CYTARABINE HYDROCHLORIDE (ARA-C)

Cytosar-U
Antimetabolite
Injection: 100 and 500 mg; 1- and 2-g vials
Pregnancy category C

Indications:

Treatment of leukemias; may be used in preconditioning regimen for bone marrow transplantation.

Dosage:

Refer to individual protocol.

Infants under 3 years: 3.3 mg/kg/day IV/SQ for 4 days

Children and adults:

Induction remission: 200 mg/m^2/day for 5 days at 2-week intervals as a single agent; 100 to 200 mg/m^2/day (or 2 to 6 mg/kg/day) for 5 to 10 days or every day until remission (combination chemotherapy). Give IV continuous infusion or every 12 hours.

Maintenance: 1 to 1.5 mg/kg IM/SQ as a single dose at 1- to 4-week intervals or 70 to 200 mg/m^2/day for 2 to 5 days at monthly intervals.

High dose cytarabine (AML, relapsed ALL) doses to 3 gm/m^2/dose.

For CNS treatment and prophylaxis (intrathecal dose): under 1 year, 20 mg; 1 to 2 years, 30 mg; 2 to 3 years, 50 mg; over 3 years, 70 mg

Contraindications:

Hypersensitivity to cytarabine. May need to reduce dose with myelosuppression or hepatic dysfunction. May cause nausea, vomiting, mucositis, fever, headache, somnolence, anorexia, alopecia, conjunctivitis, ataxia, diarrhea, hepatic dysfunction, and peripheral neuropathy. Decadron ophthalmic drops may decrease effects of conjunctivitis.

DACARBAZINE

DTIC-Dome
Antineoplastic
Injection: 100 and 200 mg
Pregnancy category C

Indications:

Treatment of Hodgkin's disease, soft-tissue sarcomas, medullary carcinoma of the thyroid, and neuroblastoma.

Dosage:

Refer to individual protocol.

Solid tumors: 200 to 470 mg/m^2/day IV over 5 days every 21 to 28 days

Neuroblastoma: 800 to 900 mg/m^2 IV as a single dose on day 1 of the cycle every 3 to 4 weeks

Hodgkin's disease: 375 mg/m^2 on days 1 and 15 of each course, repeated every 28 days

Contraindications:

Hypersensitivity to dacarbazine. Dosage reduction may be necessary in patients with renal or hepatic insufficiency. Avoid drug extravasation. Phenytoin and phenobarbital may induce dacarbazine metabolism.

DACTINOMYCIN (Actinomycin D)
Cosmegen
Antineoplastic antibiotic
Injection: 500-μg vial
Pregnancy category C

Indications:
Treatment of Wilms' tumor, rhabdomyosarcoma, and Ewing's sarcoma and other malignancies.

Dosage:
Refer to individual protocol.
Children over 6 months to adult: 15 μg/kg/day or 400 to 600 μg/m^2/day once daily for 5 days (maximum 500 μg/day); repeat every 3 to 6 weeks. Higher doses are given in some protocols.

Contraindications:
Hypersensitivity to dactinomycin. Avoid in infants under 6 months of age because of increased adverse events. Use with caution in patients with hepatobiliary dysfunction or who have received radiation (radiation recall). Reduce dosage in patients receiving concurrent radiation. Avoid extravasation. May cause myelosuppression, anorexia, vomiting, diarrhea, and stomatitis.

DAUNORUBICIN HYDROCHLORIDE
Cerubidine
Antineoplastic antibiotic
Injection: 20-mg vial
Pregnancy category D

Indications:
Treatment of leukemias.

Dosage:
Refer to individual protocol.
Infants under 3 years: 0.67 mg/kg/day IV with repeat doses
Children: 25 to 60 mg/m^2 IV with frequency dependent on protocol

Contraindications:
Hypersensitivity to daunorubicin; congestive heart failure or arrhythmias; preexisting bone marrow suppression. Reduce dosage in patients with hepatic, biliary, or renal impairment. Incompatible with sodium bicarbonate, 5-fluorouracil, heparin, and dexamethasone. May cause myelosuppression, cardiotoxicity, nausea, vomiting, alopecia, stomatitis, and pigmentation of nail beds. Irreversible myocardial toxicity may occur as total dosage approaches 550 mg/m^2 (or 450 mg/m^2 with chest irradiation). This may be an acute or late effect.

DEFEROXAMINE MESYLATE
Desferal
Heavy metal antagonist
Injection: 500 mg
Pregnancy category C

Indications:
Treatment of acute iron intoxication and chronic transfusional iron overload.

Dosage:
Chronic iron overload:
IM: 0.5 to 1 g/day
24-Hour infusion: 50 to 120 mg/kg/day (maximum 6 g/day) at a rate not to exceed 15 mg/kg/hour
SC infusion: 40 to 60 mg/kg/day over 8 to 10 hours

Contraindications:
Avoid in severe renal disease, anuria, or primary hemochromatosis. Prolonged use can result in decreased visual acuity and neurotoxicity-related auditory abnormalities. Periodic hearing and vision exams should be performed. Discontinue use in febrile patients because of increased susceptibility to infection with *Yersinia enterocolitica*. Avoid rapid IV administration because flushing, urticaria, hypotension, and shock have been reported.

DESMOPRESSION ACETATE
DDAVP, Stimate
Antihemorrhagic
Injection: 4 µg/ml (1 ml)
Solution (nasal): 1.5 mg/ml for bleeding diatheses (Stimate)
0.1 mg/ml for diabetes insipidus
Pregnancy category B

Indications:
Maintenance of hemostasis in patients with hemophilia A during surgery and postoperatively; treatment of mucosal bleeds in patients with von Willebrand disease, central diabetes insipidus, and primary nocturnal enuresis.

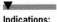

Dosage:
Von Willebrand disease and hemophilia:
IV: 0.3 μg/kg diluted in normal saline, infuse slowly over 15 to 30 minutes. Dilute in normal saline, 10 ml for children under 10 kg and 50 ml for children over 10 kg.
Intranasal administration: one puff

(150 μg) for children under 50 kg and 2 puffs (300 μg) for children over 50 kg

Peak effect is at 30 to 60 minutes, with a duration of 5 to 21 hours. Tachyphylaxis may occur with repeated doses within 72 hours.

Contraindications:
Hypersensitivity to desmopressin. Avoid in patients with severe type I, type IIB, or platelet-type von Willebrand disease and severe (<5% factor level) hemophilia. Use cautiously in patients with predisposition to thrombophilia, electrolyte imbalance, and hypertensive cardiovascular disease.

DEXAMETHASONE
Decadron
Anti-inflammatory, immune suppressant
Tablets: 0.5, 0.75, 1.5, and 4 mg
Solution: 1 mg/ml
Injection: 4 mg/ml
Pregnancy category C

Indications:
Used systemically for chronic inflammation and allergic, hematologic, neoplastic (leukemias), and autoimmune diseases; may be used in the management of cerebral edema and septic shock.

Dosage:
Antiemetic: 0.2 mg/kg/dose (5 mg/m^2/dose) 30 minutes prior to and every 6 hours after chemotherapy
Cerebral edema: loading dose: 1 to 2 mg/kg as a single dose (maximum

40 mg); maintenance: 1 to 2 mg/kg/day in 4 divided doses for 1 to 5 days, or longer
Chemotherapy: refer to individual protocol. Doses range from 6 to 20 mg/m^2/day for 5 to 7 days (may be more frequent in induction therapy).

Contraindications:
Do not administer during active, untreated infections with viral, fungal, or tuberculous organisms. Avoid in hypersensitivity. Prolonged use may cause bone pain, glucose intolerance, hypertension, and avascular necrosis of bone.

DIMERCAPROL
BAL
Antidote (chelator for gold, mercury, lead, and arsenic toxicity)
Injection: 100 mg/ml
Pregnancy category C

Indications:
Antidote to gold, mercury, and arsenic poisoning; use in conjunction with edetate calcium disodium to treat severe lead poisoning.

Dosage:
For severe lead poisoning (encephalopathy): 25 mg/kg/dose IM divided q4h for 5 to 7 days, with 50 mg/kg/day

of calcium disodium edetate as a continuous infusion beginning with second dimercaprol dose

Contraindications:
Hepatic insufficiency. Do not use in iron, selenium, or cadmium poisoning. Use with caution in patient with renal impairment or hypertension; causes hemolysis in glucose-6-phosphate dehydrogenase deficiency. Alkalinize urine.

DIPHENHYDRAMINE
Benadryl
Antihistamine
Capsules/tablets: 25 and 50 mg
Chewable tablets: 12.5 mg
Elixir: 12.5 mg/5 ml
Injection: 10 and 50 mg/ml
Pregnancy category B

Indications:
Treatment of allergic symptoms, nausea and vomiting, and motion sickness; used as an antitussive or for mild sedation. Prevents or treats phenothiazine-induced dystonic reactions.

Dosage:
Antiemetic and antivertigo: 1 mg/kg/dose every 6 hours PO, IM, or IV
Pruritus: 0.5 to 1 mg/kg/dose every 6 hours PO, IM, or IV

Contraindications:
Hypersensitivity to diphenhydramine. Use with caution in patients with glaucoma, peptic ulcer, urinary tract obstruction, and hyperthyroidism. Avoid alcohol.

Indications:
Prophylaxis and treatment of thrombo-embolic disorders such as deep vein thrombosis following surgery or trauma, and pulmonary embolus.

Dosage:
Infants under 2 months:
Prophylaxis (initial): 75 mg/kg q12h SQ
Treatment (initial): 1.5 mg/kg q12h SQ
Infants over 2 months and children 18 years or under:
Prophylaxis (initial): 0.5 mg/kg q12h SQ
Treatment (initial): 1 mg/kg q12h SQ
  Titrate dose to maintain a prophylactic range of anti–factor Xa level of 0.1 to 0.3 U/ml. For therapeutic dosing, maintain anti–factor Xa level of 0.5 to 1.0 U/ml. See text for guidelines.

  For the treatment of an acute thrombotic event, continue enoxaparin for 5 to 10 days and overlap with anticoagulation for 4 to 5 days. Alternatively, prophylaxis or treatment with enoxaparin may continue for prolonged periods (3 to 6 months) dependent on the underlying risks for thrombophilia and response to therapy.

Contraindications:
Hypersensitivity to enoxaparin or pork products (derived from porcine intestinal mucosa); active major bleeding; acute heparin-induced (or low-molecular-weight heparin–induced) thrombocytopenia; religious belief to not consume pork products.

EPOETIN ALFA (Erythropoietin)
Epogen
Blood formation
Injection: 2000, 4000, and 10,000 units
Pregnancy category C

Indications:
Treatment of anemia associated with chronic renal failure, anemia related to therapy with azathioprine in human immunodeficiency virus (HIV)–infected patients, and anemia of prematurity.

Dosage:
Usual dose is 50 to 150 U/kg administered SQ/IV three times a week.
Anemia in HIV patients: 100 U/kg/dose three times a week
Anemia in cancer patients: 150 U/kg/dose three times a week and dose titrated to effect (maximum 300 U/kg/dose)
Anemia of prematurity: 100 to 250 U/kg/dose three times a week
  A source of iron in the diet should be provided to maximize the effect of erythropoietin.

Contraindications:
Hypersensitivity to albumin; uncontrolled hypertension; neutropenia in newborns. Use with caution in patients with porphyria or a history of seizures. May cause headache and elevated blood pressure.

ETOPOSIDE (VP-16)
VePesid
Antineoplastic
Capsule: 50 mg
Injection: 20 mg/ml
Pregnancy category D

Indications:
An epipodophyllotoxin; treatment of germ cell tumors, lymphomas, brain tumors, Hodgkin's disease, leukemias, neuroblastoma, hepatoma, rhabdomyosarcoma, and histiocytosis.

Dosage:
Refer to individual protocol.
Infants: 3 mg/kg
Children: 50 to 150 mg/m^2 per protocol

Give IV infusions over at least 1 hour because of associated hypotension with rapid infusion.

Contraindications:
Hypersensitivity to etoposide. Use with caution and consider dose reduction in patients with renal impairment, hepatic impairment, or bone marrow suppression.

EUTECTIC MIXTURE OF LIDOCAINE AND PRILOCAINE
EMLA
Local anesthetic, topical anesthetic
Cream: 5- and 30-g tubes
Pregnancy category B

Indications:
Used as a topical anesthetic applied to normal intact skin to provide local anesthesia for minor procedures such as venipuncture, placement of peripheral venous access line, lumbar puncture, and minor dermatologic procedures.

Dosage:
Apply 2.5 g per site to normal intact skin and cover with occlusive dressing for 30 to 60 minutes prior to procedure.

Contraindications:
Known hypersensitivity to lidocaine, prilocaine, or other local anesthetic; methemoglobinemia. Do not use in infants under 1 month of age.

FERROUS GLUCONATE

Fergon
Iron salt
Tablet: 300 mg (35 mg elemental iron)
Elixir: 300 mg/5 ml (35 mg elemental iron/5 ml)
Pregnancy category A

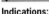
Indications:
Prevention and treatment of iron deficiency anemia.

Dosage:
(Dose is expressed in terms of elemental iron.)
Severe iron deficiency anemia: 4 to 6 mg/kg/day PO in 3 divided doses
Mild to moderate iron deficiency anemia: 3 mg/kg/day PO in 1 to 2 divided doses

Prophylaxis: 1 to 2 mg/kg/day once daily

Contraindications:
Known hypersensitivity to iron salts; hemochromatosis; transfusional iron overload. Absorption of iron is decreased when given with tetracycline, antacids, or milk. Concurrent administration of 200 mg or more of vitamin C per 30 mg elemental iron increases absorption of oral iron. May cause constipation, dark stools, nausea, and epigastric pain.

FERROUS SULFATE

Feosol, Fer-In-Sol
Iron salt
Capsule (timed release): 250 mg (50 mg elemental iron)
Tablet: 325 mg (60 to 65 mg elemental iron)
Drops: 75 mg/0.6 ml (15 mg elemental iron/0.6 ml)
Elixir: 250 mg/5 ml (44 mg elemental iron/5 ml)
Syrup: 90 mg/5 ml (18 mg elemental iron/5 ml)
Pregnancy category A

Indications:
Prevention and treatment of iron deficiency anemia.

Dosage:
See Ferrous Gluconate.

Contraindications:
See Ferrous Gluconate.

FILGRASTIM (G-CSF)
Neupogen
Blood formation
Injection: 300 µg/ml (1 ml)
Pregnancy category C

Indications:
Used to decrease the period of neutropenia and the associated risk of infection in patients with malignancies receiving myelosuppressive chemotherapy associated with a significant incidence of severe neutropenia with fever. Has been used in azathioprine-associated neutropenia in human immunodeficiency virus–infected patients and in patients with non–chemotherapy-induced neutropenia (acquired and congenital).

Dosage:
Neonates: 5 to 10 µg/kg/day IV/SQ daily for 3 to 5 days in neutropenia with sepsis
Children and adults: 5 to 10 µg/kg/day IV/SQ once daily until absolute neutrophil count (ANC) is greater than 5000 to 10,000/µl (per protocol)
Peripheral blood progenitor cell mobilization: 10 µg/kg/day SQ daily for 4 days before the first leukapheresis procedure and continued until the last leukapheresis
Congenital neutropenia: 2.5 to 6 µg/kg/day SQ; titrate according to ANC
Idiopathic or cyclic neutropenia: 5 µg/kg/day SQ once daily

Elevation of ANC is usually within 24 hours, though it may be delayed in severe myelosuppression. Transient increase in ANC may occur when granulocyte colony-stimulating factor (G-CSF) is begun shortly after completion of chemotherapy; avoid premature discontinuation.

Contraindications:
Hypersensitivity to *Escherichia coli*–derived proteins or G-CSF. *May cause bone pain and increases in uric acid and lactate dehydrogenase.*

FLUCONAZOLE
Diflucan
Antifungal
Tablet: 100 mg
Injection: 2 mg/ml
Suspension, oral: 10 mg/ml
Pregnancy category C

Indications:
Prophylaxis and treatment of susceptible fungal infections, including oropharyngeal, esophageal, and vaginal candidiasis and systemic fungal infections with *Candida*; treatment and suppression of cryptococcal meningitis. Species of *Candida* with decreased in vitro susceptibility to fluconazole are being isolated; fluconazole is more active against candidal species such as *C. albicans* than species such as *C. parapsilosis, C. glabrata*, and *C. tropicalis*.

Dosage:
Candidiasis: 6-mg/kg initial dose PO/IV, followed by 3 to 6 mg/kg/day (dependent on severity of infection) for 2 to 4 weeks (dependent on clinical response and immune status of the patient). Neonates under 14 days of age are dosed every 24 to 72 hours.
Prophylaxis in immune-compromised hosts: 3 to 6 mg/kg/dose IV/PO
IV fluconazole should be given as an infusion over 1 to 2 hours (≥6 mg/kg/day over 2 hours).

Contraindications:
Hypersensitivity to fluconazole or other azole. Antagonism may occur if amphotericin B and fluconazole are used concurrently. Many drug interactions exist, including with cyclosporine. Consult the *Physicians' Desk Reference* or a pharmacist when ordering fluconazole in a patient receiving many medications.

FOLIC ACID (Folate)
Folvite
Blood formation
Tablet: 1 mg
Injection: 5 mg/ml
Pregnancy category A/C

Indications:
Treatment of megaloblastic and macrocytic anemias resulting from folate deficiency; also used to supplement patients with chronic hemolytic anemias.

Dosage:
Recommended daily allowance (PO):
Neonates to 6 months: 35 µg
Children:
6 months to 3 years: 50 µg
4 to 6 years: 75 µg
7 to 10 years: 100 µg
11 to 14 years: 150 µg
Children over 15 years and adults:
  200 µg
Folic acid deficiency (PO, IM, IV, or SQ):
Infants: 15 µg/kg/dose daily or
  50 µg/day
Children 1 to 10 years: initial dose 1 mg/day; maintenance dose 0.1 to 0.4 mg/day
Children over 11 years and adults: initial dose 1 mg/day; maintenance dose 0.5 mg/day

Contraindications:
Pernicious, aplastic, or normocytic anemias.

GRANISETRON
Kytril
Antiemetic agent, serotonin antagonist
Tablet: 1 mg
Injection: 1 mg/ml
Pregnancy category B

Indications:
Prevention and treatment of nausea and vomiting associated with chemotherapy.

Dosage:
Children 2 years and over and adults: 20 µg/kg/dose IV 15 to 60 minutes before chemotherapy; may be repeated two to three times following chemotherapy over 24 hours. Alternatively, a single dose of 40 µg/kg/ dose 15 to 60 minutes before chemotherapy has been used.

Adults: 2 mg/24 hours PO divided q6–12h; initiate first dose before chemotherapy

Contraindications:
Inducers or inhibitors of the cytochrome P-450 drug-metabolizing enzymes may increase or decrease, respectively, the drug's clearance. Use with caution in liver disease. May cause hypertension, hypotension, arrhythmias, agitation, and insomnia.

HEPARIN SODIUM

Lipo-Hepin, Hep-Lock
Anticoagulant
Injection: many vial sizes, beef intestinal mucosa or lung origin; preservative free
Pregnancy category B

Indications:
Prophylaxis and treatment of thromboembolic disorders; prophylaxis for central venous access devices.

Dosage:
Anticoagulation in infants and children:
Initial: 50 U/kg IV bolus
Maintenance: 10 to 25 U/kg/hour as IV infusion or 50 to 100 U/kg/dose IV q4h. Adjust dose to keep partial thromboplastin time at 1.5 to 2.5 times control value
Heparin flush:
Peripheral IV: 1 to 2 ml of 10-U/ml solution q4h

Central lines: 2 to 3 ml of 100-U/ml solution q24h and after access (use 10 U/ml in neonates)
Arterial lines and total parenteral nutrition lines (central lines): add heparin to make a final concentration of 0.5 to 1 U/ml

Contraindications:
Hypersensitivity to heparin; severe thrombocytopenia; suspected intracranial hemorrhage, shock, severe hypotension, and uncontrolled bleeding (unless secondary to disseminated intravascular coagulation).

HYALURONIDASE

Wydase
Antidote (extravasation)
Injection: 150 U/ml
Pregnancy category C

Indications:
Used to influence the dispersion and absorption of other drugs, increase rate of absorption of parenteral fluids given by hypodermoclysis; treatment of IV extravasations.

Dosage:
Infants and children: Dilute 150-unit vial in 1 ml normal saline. Take 0.1 ml and dilute with 0.9 ml normal saline to yield 15 U/ml. Give 1 ml (15 units) by making five separate injections of 0.2 ml (3 units) at borders of extravasation site SQ or intradermal using a 25- or 26-gauge needle.

Contraindications:
Hypersensitivity to hyaluronidase. Do not inject in or around infected, inflamed, or cancerous lesions; do not use with dopamine or α-agonist extravasation. May cause urticaria.

HYDROCORTISONE
Hydrocortone, Solu-Cortef, Cortef, and others
Corticosteroid
Tablet (Cortef): 5, 10, and 20 mg
Injection, as sodium succinate (Solu-Cortef): 100 mg
Injection, as phosphate: 50 mg/ml
Pregnancy category C

Indications:
Treatment of inflammatory dermatoses and adrenal insufficiency; also used as a chemotherapeutic agent.

Dosage:
Physiologic replacement:
PO: 0.5 to 0.75 mg/kg/day divided q6–8h
IM: 0.25 to 0.35 mg/kg/dose qd
Anti-inflammatory/immune suppressant:
Children: 2.5 to 10 mg/kg/day PO divided q6–8h or 1 to 5 mg/kg/day IM or IV divided q12–24h

Adolescents and adults: 15 to 240 mg/dose PO, IV, or IM q12h
Intrathecal (triple intrathecal chemotherapy with methotrexate and cytarabine): dose per protocol

Contraindications:
Known hypersensitivity to hydrocortisone, polymyxin B sulfate, or neomycin sulfate. Avoid in patients with infections from herpes simplex, vaccinia, and varicella.

HYDROMORPHONE HYDROCHLORIDE
Dilaudid
Narcotic, analgesic
Tablets: 1, 2, 3, 4, and 8 mg
Liquid: 1 mg/ml
Suppository: 3 mg
Injection: 1, 2, 3, 4, and 10 mg/ml
Pregnancy category C

Indications:
Management of moderate to severe pain.

Dosage:
Children
PO: 0.03 to 0.1 mg/kg/dose q4–6h as
  needed (maximum 5 mg/dose)
IV: 0.015 mg/kg/dose q4–6h as needed
Adolescents and adults: 1 to 4 mg/
  dose PO, IV, IM, or SQ q4–6h as
  needed

Contraindications:
Hypersensitivity to hydromorphone.
Dose reduction recommended in renal
insufficiency or severe hepatic impairment. Avoid use in neonates because of potential CNS effects. Use with
caution in infants and young children.
Causes less pruritus than morphine.

HYDROXYUREA
Hydrea
Antimetabolite
Capsule: 500 mg
Pregnancy category D

Indications:
Treatment of malignancies, including
chronic myelogenous leukemia (CML);
also used as an adjunct in the management of sickle cell anemia to increase baseline hemoglobin and reduce
pain events.

Dosage:
Refer to individual protocol.
CML: initial dose is 10 to 20 mg/kg/day
  PO once daily; adjust dose according
  to hematologic response

Sickle cell anemia: initial dose is 15
  mg/kg/day (range 10 to 20 mg/kg/
  day) once daily; increase dose in increments of 5 mg/kg/day every 12
  weeks to a maximum of 35 mg/kg/day

Contraindications:
Hypersensitivity to hydroxyurea; severe
anemia and severe bone marrow
suppression. Use with caution in renal
impairment.

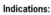

IDARUBICIN

Idamycin
Antineoplastic
Injection: 5 and 10 mg
Pregnancy category D

Indications:
Treatment of Hodgkin's disease, lymphomas, acute myelogenous leukemia, and relapsed acute lymphoblastic leukemia.

Dosage:
Refer to individual protocol. Usual dose is 5 to 12.5 mg/m^2/dose IV.

Contraindications:
Hypersensitivity to idarubicin; severe congestive heart failure or cardiomyopathy. Avoid in pre-existing bone marrow suppression unless the potential benefit warrants the risk. May need to reduce dosage in impaired renal or hepatic function. Assess cumulative dose of anthracyclines and monitor cardiac function per protocol. Irreversible myocardial toxicity may occur as total dosage approaches 550 mg/m^2 (12.5 mg idarubicin = 45 mg daunorubicin).

IFOSFAMIDE

Ifex
Alkylating agent
Injection: 1-g vial
Pregnancy category C

Indications:
Used in combination with certain other antineoplastics in the treatment of Hodgkin's disease, non-Hodgkin's lymphoma, acute lymphoblastic leukemia, osteosarcomas, rhabdomyosarcoma, Ewing's sarcoma, and advanced Wilms' tumor.

Dosage:
Refer to individual protocol. Usual dose is 700 to 1800 mg/m^2/day for 5 days.

Contraindications:
Hypersensitivity to ifosfamide. Avoid in severe bone marrow suppression. Use with caution in impaired renal function; hydrate patient prior to administration and ensure urine flow (urine specific gravity <1.010). May be used with mesna for uroprotection.

IMMUNE GLOBULIN

Gamimune N, Gammagard, Sandoglobulin, Venoglobulin, Polygam
Immunoglobulins
IV preparations: amount dependent on brand
Pregnancy category C

Indications:

Treatment of immunodeficiency states (human immunodeficiency virus [HIV]), secondary immune deficiencies (bone marrow transplant [BMT]); immune thrombocytopenic purpura (ITP), Kawasaki disease, and lymphoproliferative disorders.

Dosage:

Immunodeficiency: 200 to 400 mg/kg/dose IV every 3 to 4 weeks
Chronic lymphocytic leukemia: 400 mg/kg/dose every 3 weeks
ITP: 800 to 1000 mg/kg/day for 1 to 2 consecutive days, then every 3 to 4 weeks based on clinical response and platelet count

HIV infection: 400 mg/kg/dose every 4 weeks
HIV-associated thrombocytopenia: 500 to 1000 mg/kg/day for 1 to 5 days
Kawasaki disease: 2 g/kg as a single dose
BMT: 400 to 500 mg/kg/dose every week for 3 months, then every month (refer to protocol)

Contraindications:

Hypersensitivity to immune globulin or blood products; immunoglobulin A deficiency (except with the use of Gammagard or Polygam). May cause infusion-related toxicity and require slower IV rate and premedication with acetaminophen and diphenhydramine.

IRON DEXTRAN COMPLEX

Imferon
Iron
Injection: 50 mg elemental iron/ml (2 ml)
Pregnancy category C

Indications:
Treatment of microcytic hypochromic anemia resulting from iron deficiency in patients in whom oral administration is not feasible or is ineffective.

Dosage:
Begin with a test dose (0.5 ml [= 25 mg] or 0.25 ml [= 12.5 mg] in infants) 1 hour prior to starting iron dextran therapy.

Iron deficiency anemia: Total replacement dose of iron dextran (ml) = $0.0476 \times$ weight (kg) $\times$ (Hgb$_n$ − Hgb$_o$) + 1 ml/5 kg body weight (up to maximum of 14 ml), where

Hgb$_n$ = desired hemoglobin (g/dl) = 12 if under 15 kg or 14.8 if over 15 kg

Hgb$_o$ = measured hemoglobin (g/dl)

Acute blood loss: Total replacement dose of iron dextran (assumes 1 ml of normocytic, normochromic red cells = 1 mg elemental iron) (ml) = $0.02 \times$ blood loss (ml) $\times$ hematocrit (expressed as a decimal fraction)

Note: Total-dose infusions have been used safely and are the preferred method of administration.

Maximum daily dose, IM (injected daily or in less frequent increments):
Infants under 5 kg: 5 mg
Children 5 to 10 kg: 50 mg
Children over 10 kg and adults: 100 mg
Parenteral administration:
IM: use Z-track technique (deep into upper outer quadrant of buttock)
IV: infuse test dose over at least 5 minutes; dilute replacement dose in normal saline (50 to 100 ml) to maximum concentration of 50 mg/ml and infuse over 1 to 6 hours at a maximum rate of 50 mg/minute

Contraindications:
Hypersensitivity to iron dextran (anaphylaxis may occur); anemias not associated with iron deficiency; hemochromatosis; hemolytic anemia. Patients with underlying arthritic disease may experience an exacerbation of arthritis.
Note: Sweating, urticaria, arthralgia, fever, chills, dizziness, headache, and nausea may be delayed 24 to 48 hours after IV administration or 3 to 4 days after IM administration.

IRON COMPLEX, POLYSACCHARIDE
Niferex
Iron
Tablet: 50 mg
Capsule: 150 mg
Elixir: 100 mg/5 ml
Pregnancy category A

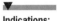

Indications:
Treatment of iron deficiency anemia.

Dosage:
See Ferrous Gluconate.

Contraindications:
See Ferrous Gluconate.

KETOROLAC TROMETHAMINE
Toradol
Nonsteroidal anti-inflammatory agent (NSAID)
Tablet: 10 mg
Injection: 15 and 30 mg/ml
Pregnancy category C

Indications:
Short-term management of pain (up to 5 days for parenteral therapy; 5 to 14 days for oral therapy).

Dosage:
Loading dose: 1 mg/kg IM; maximum dose 60 mg (loading dose not necessary in IV administration)
Maintenance dose: 0.5 mg/kg/dose IM or IV q6h; maximum dose 30 mg

Contraindications:
Hypersensitivity to ketorolac or other NSAIDs; patients with active peptic ulcer disease, gastrointestinal bleeding, or perforation; renal dysfunction; bleeding diatheses; thrombocytopenia; cerebrovascular bleeding. Use with caution in patients with congestive heart failure, hypertension, or decreased renal or hepatic function.

LEUCOVORIN CALCIUM
Wellcovorin
Antidote (anti–folic acid antagonist)
Tablets: 5, 15, and 25 mg
Injection: 50 mg, 100 mg vials
Pregnancy category C

Indications:

Antidote for folic acid antagonists (methotrexate rescue); treatment of folate-deficient megaloblastic anemias of infancy, sprue, and pregnancy; treatment of nutritional deficiencies when oral folate therapy is not possible.

Dosage:

Rescue dose: 10 mg/m^2 IV to start, then 10 mg/m^2 q6h for 72 hours; if serum creatinine 24 hours after methotrexate is elevated more than 50% or the serum methotrexate concentration is greater than 5×10^{-6} M, increase dose to 100 mg/m^2/dose q3h until serum methotrexate level is less than 1×10^{-7} M or per protocol (refer to published graphs for methotrexate clearance per protocol).

Folate-deficient megaloblastic anemia: 1 mg/day IM

Folic acid antagonist (e.g., pyrimethamine, trimethoprim) overdose: 2 to 15 mg/day PO for 3 days or until the blood counts are normal or 5 mg every 3 days; doses of 6 mg/day are needed for patients with platelet counts less than 100,000/μl.

Investigational:

Following intrathecal methotrexate: 12 mg/m^2 PO or IV as a single dose

After high-dose methotrexate: 100 to 1000 mg/m^2/dose until the serum methotrexate level is less than 1×10^{-7} M or per protocol

Contraindications:

Pernicious anemia or other megaloblastic anemias secondary to lack of vitamin B$_{12}$.

LOMUSTINE (CCNU)
CeeNU
Alkylating agent
Capsules: 10 and 40 mg
Pregnancy category D

Indications:

Treatment of brain tumors, Hodgkin's disease, and non-Hodgkin's lymphomas.

Dosage:

Refer to individual protocol. Usual dose is 75 to 150 mg/m^2 as a single dose every 6 weeks.

Contraindications:

Hypersensitivity to lomustine. May need to adjust dose because of myelosuppression. Pulmonary fibrosis may occur with high cumulative dose (>1 g/m^2).

MEPERIDINE HYDROCHLORIDE
Demerol
Narcotic, analgesic
Tablets: 50 and 100 mg
Elixir: 50 mg/5 ml
Injection: 10, 25, 50, 75, and 100 mg/ml
Pregnancy category B/D

Indications:
Management of moderate to severe pain; used as an adjunct to anesthesia and preoperative sedation.

Dosage:
Usual dose is 1 to 1.5 mg/kg/dose PO, IM, IV, or SQ q3–4h as needed; maximum dose is 100 mg.

Contraindications:
Hypersensitivity to meperidine. Avoid in patients receiving monoamine oxidase inhibitors within the past 14 days. Use with caution in renal dysfunction and seizure disorders. Accumulation of normeperidine metabolite may precipitate seizures. May cause central nervous system and respiratory depression, tachycardia, nausea, vomiting, constipation, bradycardia, hypotension, peripheral vasodilation, miosis, sedation, drowsiness, biliary or urinary tract spasm, increased intracranial pressure, and physical and psychological dependence.

MERCAPTOPURINE (6-MP)
Purinethol
Antimetabolite
Tablet: 50 mg
Pregnancy category D

Indications:
Treatment of leukemias (acute lymphoblastic, acute myelogenous, chronic myelogenous) and non-Hodgkin's lymphomas.

Dosage:
Refer to individual protocol. 75 to 100 mg/m^2 once daily

Contraindications:
Hypersensitivity to mercaptopurine; severe liver disease; severe bone marrow suppression. Use with caution and adjust dose in patients with renal or hepatic dysfunction. Patients who receive allopurinol concurrently should have their mercaptopurine dose reduced by 33%.

MESNA
Mesnex
Antidote
Injection: 100 mg/ml
Pregnancy category B

Indications:

Detoxifying agent used to inhibit hemorrhagic cystitis induced by ifosfamide and cyclophosphamide.

Dosage:

Refer to individual protocol. Dose is dependent on which antineoplastic agent it is used with.

With ifosfamide: mesna dose is 20% of ifosfamide dose 15 minutes IV before or combined with ifosfamide and 4 and 8 hours later; for high-dose ifosfamide, give dose 15 minutes before ifosfamide and every 3 hours for 3 to 6 doses. (**Note:** Total daily mesna dose ranges from 60% to 160% of the daily ifosfamide dose.)

With cyclophosphamide: mesna dose is 20% of cyclophosphamide dose given IV 15 minutes prior to cyclophosphamide dose or combined with cyclophosphamide dose and every 3 hours for 3 to 4 doses

IV continuous infusion is given with mesna doses equivalent to 60% to 100% of the ifosfamide or cyclophosphamide dose. Mesna is given by IV infusion over 15 to 30 minutes or by continuous IV infusion, or per protocol.

Contraindications:

Hypersensitivity to mesna or thiol compounds.

METHADONE HYDROCHLORIDE
Dolophine
Antidote, opioid analgesic
Tablet: 5 mg
Solution, oral: 1 mg/ml
Injection: 10 mg/ml (20 ml)
Pregnancy category B

Indications:
Management of severe pain; used in narcotic detoxification maintenance programs and for the treatment of iatrogenic narcotic dependency.

Dosage:
Children–analgesia:
IV: Initial dose is 0.1 to 0.2 mg/kg q4h for 2 to 3 doses, then q6–12h as needed; maximum 10 mg/dose
PO, IM, or SQ: Initial dose is 0.1 mg/kg q4h for 2 to 3 doses, then q6–12h as needed or 0.7 mg/kg/24 hours divided q4–6h as needed; maximum 10 mg/dose

Adults:
Analgesia: 2.5 to 10 mg PO, IM, IV, or SQ q3–8h as needed, up to 5 to 20 mg q6–8h
Detoxification: 15 to 40 mg/day PO
Maintenance of opioid dependence: 20 to 120 mg/day PO

Contraindications:
Hypersensitivity to methadone. Use with caution in patients with respiratory disease because methadone's effect on respiration (depression) lasts longer than the analgesic effects. Repeated use can result in cumulative effects, so the dose and frequency of administration may need to be reduced.

METHOTREXATE

Mexate
Antimetabolite, antineoplastic
Tablet: 2.5 mg
Injection: 50, 200, and 250 mg; 1-g vial
Pregnancy category D

Indications:
Treatment of leukemias, trophoblastic neoplasms, osteosarcoma, non-Hodgkin's lymphoma, rheumatoid arthritis, and psoriasis.

Dosage:
Refer to individual protocol.
Leukemia: 7.5 to 30 mg/m^2 once per week or every 2 weeks PO; 10 to 33,000 mg/m^2 bolus dosing or by continuous infusion over 6 to 42 hours
Osteosarcoma: 12 g/m^2 IV over 4 hours
Lymphoma: 200 to 5000 mg/m^2 IV; repeat as per protocol
Meningeal leukemia: 10 to 15 mg/m^2 intrathecally (IT) (maximum 15 mg) per protocol or
3 months or under: 3 mg
4 to 11 months: 6 mg
1 year: 8 mg
2 years: 10 mg
3 years or over: 12 to 15 mg

IT dose frequency is per protocol, dependent on treatment or prophylaxis of central nervous system leukemia
Acute lymphoblastic leukemia (relapse): loading dose of 100 mg/m^2 followed by a 35-hour infusion of 900 mg/m^2/day
Trophoblastic neoplasms: 15 to 30 mg/day PO or IM for 5 days; repeat in 7 days for 3 to 5 courses

Contraindications:
Hypersensitivity to methotrexate; severe renal or hepatic impairment; pre-existing profound bone marrow suppression. High-dose methotrexate (>1 g/m^2) should not be administered to patients with a creatinine clearance of less than 50% to 75% of normal. Patients should receive alkaline fluids to maintain urine pH of 7 or higher while receiving high-dose methotrexate. Follow serum levels per protocol and leucovorin rescue per protocol; follow methotrexate degradation curve per protocol.

METHYLPREDNISOLONE

Depo-Medrol, Solu-Medrol
Corticosteroid
Tablets: 2, 4, 8, 16, 24, and 32 mg
Injection, sodium succinate (Solu-Medrol): 40, 125, 500, 1000, and 2000 mg (IV/IM)
Pregnancy category C

Indications:

Anti-inflammatory or immune-suppressant agent used to treat a variety of diseases of hematologic, allergic, inflammatory, neoplastic, and autoimmune origin.

Dosage:

Anti-inflammatory/immune suppressant: 0.5 to 1.7 mg/kg/24 hours PO, IM, or IV divided q6–12h

Chemotherapy: Refer to individual protocols for dosing (in lieu of predni-sone; convert dose for steroid potency).

Contraindications:

Hypersensitivity to methylprednisolone. Do not administer with live-virus vaccines or during active infection with varicella or herpes zoster. Avoid use in patients with systemic fungal infections. May cause hypertension, glucose intolerance, gastrointestinal bleeding, osteoporosis, pseudotumor cerebri, and Cushing's syndrome.

METOCLOPROMIDE

Reglan
Antiemetic
Tablets: 5 and 10 mg
Syrup: 5 mg/5 ml
Injection: 5 mg/ml
Pregnancy category B

Indications:

Treatment of gastroesophageal reflux (GER) and prevention of nausea and vomiting associated with chemotherapy.

Dosage:

GER or gastrointestinal (GI) dysmotility: 0.1 to 0.2 mg/kg/dose up to QID PO, IV, or IM; maximum dose is 0.8 mg/kg/24 hours

Antiemetic: 1 to 2 mg/kg/dose q2–6h PO, IV, or IM. Premedicate with diphenhydramine to reduce extrapyramidal symptoms.

Contraindications:

Hypersensitivity to metoclopramide; GI obstruction; pheochromocytomas; history of seizure disorder. Sedation, headache, anxiety, and diarrhea may occur.

MORPHINE SULFATE

Astramorph/PF, Duramorph, MS Contin
Narcotic, Analgesic
Tablets: 15 and 30 mg
Controlled-release tablets: 15, 30, 60, and 100 mg
Sustained-release tablets: 30, 60, and 100 mg
Solution, oral: 10, 20, and 100 mg/5 ml
Suppository: 5, 10, 20, and 30 mg
Injection: 0.5, 1, 2, 3, 4, 5, 8, 10, 15, and 25 mg/ml
Pregnancy category B/D

Indications:

Relief of moderate to severe pain, acute and chronic, after non-narcotic analgesics have failed; preanesthetic medication; relief of dyspnea of acute left ventricular failure and pulmonary edema.

Dosage:

Dose should be titrated to effect.
Neonates: 0.1 to 0.2 mg/kg IV q3–4h; q6h dosing may be appropriate for extremely premature infants or infants with hepatic dysfunction
Infants and children:
Tablet and solution (prompt release): 0.2 to 0.5 mg/kg/dose PO q4–6h as needed
Tablet (controlled release): 0.3 to 0.6 mg/kg/dose PO q12h
0.05 to 0.1 mg/kg/dose IM, IV, or SQ q2–4h as needed; maximum 15 mg/dose

Sickle cell or cancer pain: 0.025 to 2.6 mg/kg/hour IV or SQ continuous infusion
Sedation/analgesia for procedures: 0.05 to 0.1 mg/kg IV 5 minutes prior to procedure (maximum 3 to 4 mg/dose)
Patient-controlled analgesia (PCA) dosing guidelines:
PCA dose: 0.01 to 0.03 mg/kg
Continuous dose: 0.01 mg/kg/hour
Bolus (loading): 0.03 to 0.1 mg/kg
One-hour maximum is 0.1 mg/kg/hour (6 to 8 mg/hour)

Contraindications:

Hypersensitivity to morphine sulfate; increased intracranial pressure; severe respiratory depression; severe renal or liver insufficiency. May cause severe pruritus, urinary retention, respiratory depression, central nervous system depression, constipation, and ileus. Prolonged use can result in physical and psychological dependence.

NALOXONE

Narcan
Opioid antagonist
Injection: 0.4 and 1 mg/ml
Pregnancy category B

Indications:

Used to reverse central nervous system and respiratory depression in suspected narcotic overdose; treatment of coma of unknown etiology.

Dosage:

Note: The dose for pediatric postoperative narcotic reversal is **one tenth** of the dose for opiate intoxication.

Premature infant to 5 years or under 20 kg: 0.1 mg/kg; repeat every 2 to 3 minutes if needed. May need to repeat doses every 20 to 60 minutes.

Over 5 years or 20 kg or over: 2 mg/ dose; if no response, repeat every 2 to 3 minutes. May need to repeat doses every 20 to 60 minutes.

Children and adults: IV continuous infusion. Calculate the initial dosage per hour based on the effective intermittent dose used and duration of adequate response seen; titrate dose to a range of 2.5 to 160 µg/kg/hour

Patient-controlled analgesia side effect reversal (pruritus with morphine): IV continuous infusion. Begin with 1 µg/kg/hour; taper infusion gradually over 2 to 4 hours.

Endotracheal administration can be done safely by diluting in 1 to 2 ml of normal saline.

Contraindications:

Hypersensitivity to naloxone.

ONDANSETRON

Zofran
Antiemetic, Serotonin antagonist
Tablets: 4 and 8 mg
Injection: 2 mg/ml (2 ml, 20 ml)
Pregnancy category B

Indications:

Prevention of nausea and vomiting associated with initial and repeat courses of emetogenic cancer chemotherapy and prevention of postoperative nausea and vomiting.

Dosage:

Prevention of chemotherapy-induced nausea and vomiting:

IV: 0.15 mg/kg/dose 30 minutes prior to the start of emetogenic chemotherapy, with subsequent doses administered 4 and 8 hours after the first dose or every 8 hours until chemotherapy is complete for a maximum of 24 hours after completion of chemotherapy. Alternatively (for highly emetogenic drugs), give 0.45 mg/kg/24 hours as a single dose 30 minutes prior to start of chemotherapy. Maximum single dose 24 mg.

Oral: Dose based on body surface area or age:

Less than 0.3 m²: 1 mg TID
0.3 to 0.6 m²: 2 mg TID
0.6 to 1 m²: 3 mg TID
Greater than 1 m²: 4 to 8 mg TID
Age 4 to 12 years: 4 mg two to three times a day; first dose 30 minutes prior to start of chemotherapy
Children over 12 years and adults: 8 mg two to three times a day; first dose 30 minutes prior to start of chemotherapy

Contraindications:

Hypersensitivity to ondansetron. Ondansetron is metabolized by the cytochrome P-450 enzyme system, so inducers or inhibitors of this system may affect the elimination of ondansetron. Data are limited for use in children under 3 years of age. May need to adjust dose and interval for severe hepatic impairment. Side effects are usually mild, with headache, sedation, constipation, and dry mouth being the most common.

PEGASPARGASE (PEG-L-Asparaginase)
Oncaspar
Antineoplastic
Injection: 750 U/ml
Pregnancy category C

Indications:
Induction treatment of acute lympho-blastic leukemia (ALL) in combination with other chemotherapeutic agents; also given in other phases of therapy and in relapsed ALL; treatment of acute myelogenous leukemia and lymphomas.

Dosage:
Refer to individual protocol. Usual dose is 2500 U/m^2 IM every 14 days or per protocol.

Patients should be observed in the clinic or hospital setting for a minimum of 1 hour after administration of L-asparaginase.

Contraindications:
Prior allergic reaction to pegaspargase; pancreatitis; prior significant hemor-rhagic event with asparaginase. Use with caution in patients with hepatic im-pairment or receiving other hepatotoxic drugs; use with caution in patients receiving anticoagulation, aspirin, or nonsteroidal anti-inflammatory drugs. May have drug interactions with metho-trexate, vincristine, and highly protein-bound drugs. May cause hyperglycemia, hyperuricemia, hyperammonemia, hemorrhagic cystitis, decreased fibrino-gen, thrombosis, hemorrhage, and anaphylaxis. Decadron may help allevi-ate allergic symptoms.

PENTAMIDINE ISETHIONATE
Pentam 300, NebuPent
Antibiotic, antiprotozoal
Injection: 300-mg vial
Aerosol: 300-mg vial
Pregnancy category C

Indications:
Treatment of *Pneumocystis carinii* pneu-monia (PCP) in patients who cannot tolerate or who fail to respond to trime-thoprim–sulfamethoxazole; prevention of PCP in immune compromised hosts; treatment of African trypanosomiasis; treatment of visceral leishmaniasis caused by *Leishmania donovani*.

Dosage:
Prophylaxis for PCP:
IM/IV: 4 mg/kg/dose every 2 to 4 weeks
Inhalation (≥5 years): 300 mg in 6 ml
   H$_2$O via inhalation every month
   (Respirgard II nebulizer)

Maximum single dose is 300 mg.
Treatment of PCP: 4 mg/kg/dose IM/IV qd × 14 to 21 days

Contraindications:
Hypersensitivity to pentamidine isethion-ate. Adjust dose in renal impairment. Use with caution in patients with diabe-tes mellitus, renal or hepatic dysfunc-tion, hypertension, or hypotension. Addi-tive toxicity is seen with amphotericin B, cisplatin, vancomycin, and didanosine. Can see Jarisch-Herxheimer–like reaction. Inhalation therapy may cause irritation of the airway.

PREDNISONE
Deltasone, Meticorten, Orasone
Glucocorticoid, immune suppressant
Tablets: 1, 2, 5, 10, 20, and 50 mg
Solution: 1 and 5 mg/ml
Pregnancy category C

Indications:
Management of adrenocortical insufficiency; used for anti-inflammatory or immune suppressant effects and as chemotherapy.

Dosage:
Dose is dependent on condition being treated and response of patient. Consider alternate-day therapy for long-term therapy. Discontinuation of long-term therapy requires gradual tapering.
Anti-inflammatory or immune suppressant (includes immune thrombocytopenic purpura, aplastic anemia): 0.05 to 4 mg/kg/day PO divided one to four times a day
Chemotherapy: 40 to 180 mg/m^2/day or as per protocol

Physiologic replacement: 4 to 5 mg/m^2/day

Contraindications:
Serious infections, except septic shock or tuberculous meningitis; systemic fungal infections; varicella; hypersensitivity to prednisone. Use with caution in patients with hypothyroidism, cirrhosis, hypertension, congestive heart failure, ulcerative colitis, gastrointestinal bleeding, and thromboembolic disorders. May cause hypertension, hyperglycemia, irritability, gastritis, skin atrophy, osteoporosis, cataracts, fluid retention, and weight gain. Consider use of antacid in long-term therapy.

PROCARBAZINE HYDROCHLORIDE
Matulane
Alkylating agent
Capsule: 50 mg
Pregnancy category D

FORMULARY

Indications:
Treatment of Hodgkin's disease, non-Hodgkin's lymphoma, and brain tumors.

Dosage:
Refer to individual protocol. Usual dose is 50 to 100 mg/m^2 PO daily for 10 to 14 days.

Contraindications:
Hypersensitivity to procarbazine; pre-existing bone marrow aplasia. Use with caution and reduce dose in patients with renal or hepatic impairment or marrow suppression. May potentiate central nervous system depression when used with phenothiazine derivatives, barbiturates, narcotics, alcohol, tricyclic antidepressants, and methyldopa. Drug (monoamine oxidase inhibitors) and food interactions are common. Avoid food with high tyramine content (cheese, tea, dark beer, coffee, cola drinks, wine, and bananas) because hypertensive crisis, tremor, excitation, cardiac palpitations, and angina may occur.

RH$_0$ (D) IMMUNE GLOBULIN (IV)
WinRho SD
Immune globulin
Injection: 600 and 1500 IU (1 µg = 5 IU)
Pregnancy category C

Indications:
Treatment of immune thrombocytopenic purpura (ITP) in nonsplenectomized Rh$_0$(D)-positive patients.

Dosage:
Hemoglobin of 10 g/dl or greater: 250 IU/kg/dose IV once
Hemoglobin less than 10 g/dl: 125 to 200 IU/kg/dose IV once
Additional doses: 125 to 300 IU/kg/dose IV; actual dose and frequency are determined by the patient's response. Administer dose over 3 to 5 minutes.

WinRho SD is currently the only Rh$_0$(D) immune globulin product compatible with IV administration.

Contraindications:
Known hypersensitivity to immune globulins or thimerosal; patients with immunoglobulin A deficiency. Use with extreme caution in patients with a hemoglobin less than 8 g/dl. Adverse events associated with ITP include headache, chills, fever, and reduction in hemoglobin (resulting from the destruction of Rh$_0$(D) antigen–positive cells). May interfere with immune response to live-virus vaccines.

SARGRAMOSTIM (GM-CSF)

Leukine, Prokine
Colony-stimulating factor
Injection: 250 and 500 µg
Pregnancy category C

Indications:

Used for myeloid reconstitution after autologous bone marrow transplant (BMT); to accelerate myeloid recovery in patients with non-Hodgkin's lymphoma, Hodgkin's lymphoma, and acute lymphoblastic leukemia undergoing autologous BMT; and to accelerate myeloid engraftment following chemotherapy.

Dosage:

Usual dose is 250 µg/m^2/day IV over at least 2 hours. Administer daily until the absolute neutrophil count is 5000/µl or greater for 1 day or until day +21 post-BMT, whichever comes first (or per protocol).

Do not administer within 24 hours prior to or after chemotherapy or 12 hours prior to radiation therapy.

Contraindications:

Excessive leukemic myeloid blasts in the peripheral blood or bone marrow (≥10%); history of immune thrombocytopenic purpura; known hypersensitivity to granulocyte-macrophage colony-stimulating factors or yeast-derived products. Use with caution in patients with autoimmune or chronic inflammatory conditions, hypertension, cardiovascular disease, pulmonary disease, or renal or hepatic impairment.

SUCCIMER

Chemet (2,3-dimercaptosuccinic acid; DMSA)
Antidote (chelator for lead toxicity)
Capsule: 100 mg
Pregnancy category C

Indications:

Treatment of lead poisoning in asymptomatic children with blood levels greater than 45 µg/dl.

Dosage:

Usual dose is 30 mg/kg/day PO divided q8h for 5 days, followed by 20 mg/kg/day PO divided q12h for 14 days.

Repeat courses separated by a minimum of 2 weeks may be necessary to treat rebound lead concentrations (resulting from mobilization of lead from bone stores).

Contraindications:

Known hypersensitivity to succimer. Use with caution in impaired renal function.

SULFAMETHOXAZOLE AND TRIMETHOPRIM

Bactrim, Bactrim DS, Septra, Septra DS
Antibiotic, sulfonamide derivative
Tablet, single strength: 400 mg sulfamethoxazole (SMX) and 80 mg
    trimethoprim (TMP)
Tablet, double strength: 800 mg SMX and 160 mg TMP
Suspension, oral: 200 mg SMX/40 mg TMP per 5 ml
Injection: 80 mg SMX/ml and 16 mg TMP/ml
Pregnancy category C

Indications:

Oral treatment of urinary tract infections
(UTIs) and otitis media; prophylaxis of
Pneumocystis carinii pneumonitis (PCP);
IV treatment of documented PCP and
empiric treatment of suspected PCP
in immune compromised patients; treatment of documented or suspected
shigellosis, typhoid fever, or *Nocardia
asteroides* infections.

Dosage:

(Dosage recommendations are based on
the TMP component.)
    May be given PO or IV.
Neonates: restricted
Children over 2 months:
Minor infection: 6 to 10 mg TMP/kg/day
    PO divided q12h
Serious infection/PCP: 15 to 20 mg
    TMP/kg/day divided q6h
UTI or otitis media prophylaxis: 2 mg
    TMP/kg once daily
Prophylaxis for PCP: 5 mg TMP/kg/day
    divided q12h two to three times a
week (maximum dose 320 to 960 mg
TMP/day)

Contraindications:

Hypersensitivity to sulfa drug or any
component; porphyria; megaloblastic
anemia due to folate deficiency. Do not
use in infants under 2 months of age.
Use with caution in patients with
glucose-6-phosphate dehydrogenase deficiency and impaired renal or hepatic
impairment. Serious adverse reactions include Stevens-Johnson syndrome, toxic epidermal necrolysis, hepatic necrosis, agranulocytosis, aplastic
anemia, and other blood dyscrasias. Discontinue with rash. May need to be held
temporarily in oncology patients (PCP
prophylaxis) who develop neutropenia.
Numerous drug interactions are reported. SMX-TMP decreases the clearance of warfarin and methotrexate,
decreases serum cyclosporine concentrations, and increases the effect of sulfonylureas, phenytoin, and thiopental.

THIOGUANINE (6-TG)

Antimetabolite
Tablet: 40 mg
Pregnancy category D

Indications:

Remission induction in acute myelogenous leukemia; treatment of chronic myelogenous leukemia and acute lymphoblastic leukemia.

Dosage:

Refer to individual protocol.
Infants under 3 years: 3.3 mg/kg/day PO divided q12h for 4 days
Children and adults: 2 to 3 mg/kg/day PO (calculated to nearest 20 mg) or 50 to 200 mg/m^2/day PO divided q12–24h for 4 to 7 days or per protocol

Contraindications:

Hypersensitivity to thioguanine. Use with caution and reduce dosage in patients with renal or hepatic impairment. May cause nausea or vomiting, anorexia, stomatitis, diarrhea, myelosuppression, and veno-occlusive disease. Increases busulfan toxicity.

THIOTEPA

Thioplex
Alkylating agent
Powder for injection: 15 mg
Pregnancy category D

Indications:

Treatment of superficial tumors of the bladder, lymphomas and sarcomas, and meningeal neoplasms; control of pleural, pericardial, or peritoneal effusions caused by metastatic tumors; also used in high-dose regimens with autologous bone marrow transplantation (ABMT).

Dosage:

Refer to individual protocol.
Sarcomas: 25 to 65 mg/m^2 IV as a single dose every 3 to 4 weeks

ABMT: 300 mg/m^2/dose over 3 hours IV; repeat q24h for 3 doses. Maximum tolerated dose over 3 days is 900 to 1125 mg/m^2

Contraindications:

Hypersensitivity to thiotepa; severe myelosuppression. Reduce dose in patients with renal, hepatic, or bone marrow dysfunction. May cause central nervous system changes, skin hyperpigmentation, nausea and vomiting, hematuria, and elevation of liver transaminases and bilirubin.

THROMBIN, TOPICAL

Hemostatic agent, blood product
Powder: 1000- and 5000-unit vial; 10,000- and 20,000-unit kit
Pregnancy category C

Indications:

Hemostasis where minor bleeding from capillaries and small venules is accessible.

Dosage:

Apply powder directly to the site of bleeding or on oozing surface, or use 1000 to 2000 U/ml of solution where bleeding is profuse. Use 100 U/ml for bleeding from skin or mucosal surfaces.

Contraindications:

Hypersensitivity to thrombin or material of bovine origin. May cause fever or allergic reactions. Topical use only.

TRANEXAMIC ACID

Cyklokapron
Antihemophilic agent
Tablet: 500 mg
Injection: 100 mg/ml
Pregnancy category D

Indications:

Short-term use (2 to 8 days) in hemophilia or von Willebrand disease patients for mucosal bleeding (including tooth extraction) to reduce or prevent hemorrhage.

Dosage:

IV: 10 mg/kg immediately before oral surgery, followed by oral therapy
PO: 25 mg/kg/dose q6–8h for 2 to 8 days

Contraindications:

Subarachnoid hemorrhage; active intravascular clotting process; acquired defective color vision. Use with caution in patients with renal impairment or cardiovascular or cerebrovascular disease. Dose modification is required in patients with renal impairment. May cause hypotension, thromboembolic complications, headache, and visual abnormalities (animals).

URATE OXIDASE

Rasburicase
Hyperuricemic agent (enzyme)
Injection: 1.5 mg/3 ml vials

Indications:

Short-term management or prevention of hyperuricemia in patients with leukemia or lymphoma.

Not currently approved by the Food and Drug Administration; available only on a compassionate-use basis.

Dosage:

Usual dose is 0.2 mg/kg in 50 ml preservative-free normal saline IV over 30 minutes, repeat q12–24h as needed up to 3 to 7 days.

Give prior to chemotherapy in expected massive tumor lysis.

Contraindications:

Hypersensitivity to urate oxidase; glucose-6-phosphate dehydrogenase deficiency (may cause hemolytic anemia); severe asthma. May cause rash, headache, or bronchospasm.

UROKINASE

Abbokinase, Abbokinase Open-Cath
Thrombolytic enzyme
Injection: 5000 U/ml (Open Cath); 250,000 units (preservative free)
Pregnancy category B

Indications:

Treatment of recent severe or massive arterial or deep venous thrombosis (DVT), pulmonary embolus (PE), or occluded central lines.

Dosage:

DVT or PE: 4400 U/kg IV over 10 minutes, followed by 4400 U/kg/hour for 12 to 72 hours; titrate to effect (doses as high as 10,000 U/kg/hour have been used)

Occluded catheter:

Instillation: instill 5000 U/ml into each lumen of the catheter, allow to dwell 1 hour, then aspirate; may repeat with 5000 or 10,000 U/ml in each lumen if no response

IV infusion: 150 to 200 U/kg/hour in each lumen for 8 to 48 hours at a rate of at least 20 ml/hour

Monitor clot q12–24h for response.

Contraindications:

Hypersensitivity to urokinase; internal bleeding; cerebrovascular accident within 2 months; brain tumor, arteriovenous malformation, or history of aneurysm; recent (within 10 days) trauma or surgery; bacterial endocarditis. Discontinue if bleeding occurs or patient develops rash, fever, or allergic symptoms. Monitor coagulation studies (prothrombin time, activated partial thromboplastin time, and fibrinogen) before and during continuous administration.

VINBLASTINE SULFATE
Velban
Antineoplastic
Injection: 10-mg vial
Pregnancy category D

Indications:
Treatment of Hodgkin's disease, histiocytosis, choriocarcinoma, advanced testicular tumors, and non-Hodgkin's lymphomas.

Dosage:
Refer to individual protocol.
Hodgkin's disease: 1.5 to 6 mg/m²/ dose IV once every 1 to 4 weeks for three to six cycles
Histiocytosis: 0.4 mg/kg/dose IV once every 7 to 10 days
Germ cell tumors: 0.2 mg/kg IV on days 1 and 2 of each cycle every 3 weeks for four cycles

Contraindications:
Hypersensitivity to vinblastine; severe leukopenia. Dose modification may be needed in patients with hepatic impairment or neurotoxicity. Avoid extravasation. May cause peripheral neuropathy, myelosuppression, jaw pain, myalgia, paresthesia, constipation, abdominal pain, ileus, and mild alopecia.
Intrathecal administration may cause death.

VINCRISTINE SULFATE
Oncovin
Antineoplastic
Injection: 1- and 2-mg vials (1 mg/ml)
Pregnancy category D

Indications:
Treatment of leukemias, Hodgkin's disease, neuroblastoma, malignant lymphomas, Wilms' tumor, and rhabdomyosarcoma.

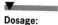

Dosage:
Refer to individual protocol.
Children 10 kg or under or body surface area (BSA) less than 1 m²: 0.05 mg/kg IV once weekly; maximum single dose 2 mg
Children over 10 kg or BSA 1 m² or greater: 1 to 2 mg/m² IV; may repeat weekly for 3 to 6 weeks. Maximum single dose is 2 mg.
Neuroblastoma: IV continuous infusion with doxorubicin: 0.66 to 1 mg/m²/day for 72 hours
The maximum dose may exceed 2 mg for the treatment of Hodgkin's disease (refer to protocol).

Contraindications:
Hypersensitivity to vincristine. Avoid in patients with the demyelinating form of Charcot-Marie-Tooth disease. Asparaginase may decrease clearance of vincristine. Dose modification may be required in patients with impaired hepatic function, pre-existing neuromuscular disease, or severe side effects of treatment with vincristine. Avoid extravasation. May cause peripheral neuropathy, paresthesias, ileus, jaw pain, cranial nerve paralysis (ptosis), syndrome of inappropriate antidiuretic hormone secretion, alopecia, and constipation.
Intrathecal administration may cause death.

VITAMIN K₁/PHYTONADIONE
AquaMEPHYTON, Mephyton
Vitamin, water soluble
Tablet: 5 mg
Injection: 2 and 10 mg/ml
Pregnancy category C

Indications:
Prevention and treatment of hypoprothrombinemia caused by anticoagulants or drug-induced vitamin K deficiency and of hemorrhagic disease of the newborn.

Dosage:
Hemorrhagic disease of the newborn:
Prophylaxis: 0.5 to 1 mg IM/SQ within 1 hour of birth; may repeat 6 to 8 hours later if necessary
Treatment: 1 to 2 mg/dose IM/SQ per day
Oral anticoagulant overdose:
Infants: 1 to 2 mg/dose IM, IV, or SQ q4–8h

Children and adults:
2.5 to 10 mg/dose IM, IV, or SQ; may repeat in 6 to 8 hours
2.5 to 10 mg/dose PO; may repeat in 12 to 48 hours
Vitamin K deficiency (due to drugs, malabsorption, or decreased synthesis of vitamin K by the liver): 2.5 to 5 mg/24 hours PO or 1 to 2 mg/dose IM, IV, or SQ as a single dose (up to 10 mg in adults)

Contraindications:
Hypersensitivity to phytonadione. Antagonizes action of warfarin.

WARFARIN SODIUM
Coumadin
Anticoagulants
Tablets: 1, 2, 2.5, 3, 4, 5, 6, 7.5, and 10 mg
Injection: 2 mg/ml
Pregnancy category D

Indications:
Prophylaxis and treatment of venous thromboembolic disorders; prevention of arterial thromboembolism in patients with prosthetic heart valves or atrial fibrillation; prevention of death, venous thromboembolism, and recurrent myocardial infarction (MI) after acute MI.

Dosage:
Infants and children (to maintain an International Normalized Ratio [INR] between 2 and 3):
Initial dose: 0.2 mg/kg PO for 1 to 2 days; maximum dose 10 mg
Maintenance dose: 0.1 mg/kg/24 hours PO daily; range 0.05 to 0.34 mg/kg/24 hours

Onset of action is within 36 to 72 hours and peak effects occur within 5 to 7 days. Monitor INR after 5 to 7 days of new dosage.

Usual duration of therapy for first venous thrombotic event is 3 months.

Contraindications:
Hypersensitivity to warfarin; severe liver or kidney disease; uncontrolled bleeding; gastrointestinal (GI) ulcers; neurosurgical procedures; malignant hypertension. Concomitant use with vitamin K may decrease anticoagulant effect. Concomitant use with aspirin, nonsteroidal anti-inflammatory drugs, or indomethacin may increase warfarin's anticoagulant effect and cause severe GI irritation. May cause fever, skin lesions, necrosis (especially in protein C deficiency), hemorrhage, hemoptysis, anorexia, nausea, vomiting, and diarrhea. Many drug interactions exist; review all medications prior to initiation of therapy. Antidote is vitamin K and fresh frozen plasma.

REFERENCES

Wemmer J (ed). Drug Formulary Children's Hospital Oakland, 3rd ed. Hudso, OH: Lexi-Comp., Inc., 2002.

Skeel RT (ed). Handbook of Cancer Chemotherapy, 5th ed. Baltimore: Lippincott–Williams & Wilkins, 1999.

Physicians' Desk Reference, 55th ed. Montvale, NJ: Medical Economics Company, Inc., 2001.

INDEX

Note: Page numbers followed by f refer to figures; page numbers followed by t refer to tables.

A

Abdominal mass
  evaluation of, 124–125
  in neuroblastoma, 187
Abdominal pain, 154–155
Acetaminophen, in nonhemolytic transfusion reaction, 58t
Activated partial thromboplastin time, 69–70, 71t
Activated prothrombin complex concentrates, in hemophilia A, 88
Acute chest syndrome, in sickle cell disease, 26–29, 29f
Acute lymphoblastic leukemia, 161–166, 162t
  clinical presentation of, 161–162, 162t
  complications of, 165
  diagnosis of, 162t, 163
  relapse of, 165–166
  risk group classification of, 164
  treatment of, 164–165
Acute myelogenous leukemia, 166–168, 166t
  classification of, 166, 166t, 167
  clinical presentation of, 166–167
  complications of, 168
  diagnosis of, 167
  relapse of, 168
  treatment of, 167–168
Acyclovir, 149, 204
Adriamycin, 133t, 221
Alkalinization, in hyperleukocytosis, 156
Allergic reaction, transfusion-related, 57

Alloimmune thrombocytopenia, neonatal, 113–115
Alloimmunization, transfusion-related, 59
Allopurinol, 205
  in hyperleukocytosis, 156
  in tumor lysis syndrome, 158
Alteplase, 143, 206
Amegakaryocytic thrombocytopenia, congenital, 118
Amifostine, 207
Aminocaproic acid, 207
  in hemophilia-related hemorrhage, 87–88
  in von Willebrand disease, 77
Amphotericin B, 151, 208
  liposomal, 210
Amphotericin B cholesteryl sulfate, 209
Amphotericin B lipid complex, 209
Analgesia, in sickle cell disease, 24–26
Anemia, 1–10
  erythropoietin in, 8–9
  evaluation of, 2–6, 2f, 3t, 4t–5t, 6f, 7f
  Fanconi's, 118
  hemoglobin in, 6f
  hemolytic, 11–17
    evaluation of, 14–16, 15f
    in red cell enzyme defects, 12–14
    in red cell membrane disorders, 11–12
    treatment of, 16–17
  in sickle cell disease, 32–33
  iron deficiency, 1–2, 6–10
  medical history in, 4t–5t

Anemia *(Continued)*
  oral iron challenge in, 7–8
  oral iron therapy in, 6–7
  parenteral iron therapy in, 8
  physical examination in, 5t
  transfusion therapy in, 9–10
Antibiotics
  in acute chest syndrome,
    28, 29f
  prophylactic, 127–128
Anticoagulation therapy,
  in venous thrombosis,
    95, 97–100
Antiemetics, 131–135, 134t
α_2-Antiplasmin deficiency, 81
Antithrombin III
  deficiency of, 94, 94t
  therapeutic, 54
Antiviral agents, prophylactic,
  128–130, 129t
Aplastic crisis, in sickle cell
  disease, 33
ARA-C, 132t, 134t, 215–216
Asparaginase, 133t, 210
Aspergillus infection, prevention of,
  130–131
Astrocytoma, 174–175
Avascular necrosis, in sickle cell
  disease, 33–34

B

Bacterial endocarditis, prophylactic
  antibiotics for, 128
Bernard-Soulier syndrome, 118
Biopsy, bone marrow, 193–195
  in neuroblastoma, 125, 188
  in non-Hodgkin's lymphoma, 181
Bleeding disorders, 67–72
  activated partial thromboplastin
    time in, 69–70, 71t
  acute hemorrhage in, 83–91.
    See also Hemorrhage.
  fibrinogen in, 70
  hemoglobin in, 68
  International Normalized Ratio
    in, 69

Bleeding disorders *(Continued)*
  laboratory evaluation in, 68–72,
    71t, 72f
  patient history in, 67, 68t
  physical examination in, 68
  platelet count in, 69, 71t
  prothrombin time in, 69, 71t
  thrombin time in, 70
Bleomycin sulfate, 133t,
  134t, 211
Blood transfusion, 47–55.
  See also Transfusion therapy.
Body surface area, 129t
Bone marrow
  aspiration of, 193–195
    in acute lymphocytic leuke-
      mia, 163
    in acute myelogenous leuke-
      mia, 167
    in brain tumor, 172
    in suspected leukemia, 123
  biopsy of, 193–195
  replacement of, neutropenia
    with, 102
  transplantation of, 167–168
Bone pain, 120t, 122
  in acute lymphoblastic leuke-
    mia, 162
Bone scan, 172, 184, 189
Brain
  astrocytoma of, 174–175
  ependymoma of, 175
  medulloblastoma of, 173–174
  tumors of, 171–175
    clinical presentation of,
      171–172
    diagnosis of, 172
    treatment of, 173
Busulfan, 211

C

Calcium disodium edetate, in lead
  toxicity, 65, 222
Cancer
  abdominal mass in, 124–125
  bone pain in, 120t, 122

Cancer *(Continued)*
  evaluation of, 119–125
  fever in, 145–152, 146f
  headache in, 119, 121t
  hyperleukocytosis in, 120t, 122
  lymphadenopathy in,
      120–121, 120t
  pancytopenia in, 120t, 122
  presentation of, 119–122, 121t
  supportive care in, 127–138
    antiemetics for, 131–135,
      132t–133t, 134t
    hematopoietic growth factors
      for, 135–138
    infection prevention for,
      127–131, 129t, 130t
    oral hygiene for, 127
Cannabinoids, for vomiting, 135
Carboplatin, 132t, 134t, 212
Carmustine, 212
Catheter, central venous, 141–143
  infection with, 148–149
  thromboembolism with, 93–94
CCNU, 236
Central nervous system. *See also*
      Brain.
  in acute lymphoblastic leuke-
      mia, 162
Cerebral vascular disease, in sickle
      cell disease, 19–20
Cerebrovascular accident, in sickle
      cell disease, 30–32
Chelation therapy, 61–65
  in iron overload, 61–62
  in lead toxicity, 62–65
Chemotherapy, 132t–133t
  extravasations of, 197–198,
      197t
  in acute lymphoblastic leukemia,
      164–165
  in acute myelogenous leukemia,
      167–168
  in brain tumor, 173
  in Hodgkin's disease, 179
  in neuroblastoma, 190
  in non-Hodgkin's lymphoma,
      181–182

Chemotherapy *(Continued)*
  in superior vena cava
      syndrome, 154
  into Ommaya reservoir, 193
  intrathecal, 191–192
  peripheral administration of,
      195–196
  vomiting with, 131–135,
      134t
Chest radiography, in sickle cell
      disease, 27
Chlorhexidine mouth rinse, 127
Chronic benign neutropenia,
      101–102
Cisplatin, 132t, 134t, 213
Clotrimazole, oral, 130
Computed tomography
  in brain tumor, 172
  in neuroblastoma, 189
Congenital amegakaryocytic
      thrombocytopenia, 118
Corticosteroids, in immune
      thrombocytopenic purpura,
      112–113
Cryoprecipitate, 53–54
Cyclophosphamide, 132t,
      134t, 214
Cyclosporine, 215
Cytarabine hydrochloride, 132t,
      134t, 215–216
Cytomegalovirus infection,
      129, 149
  pretransfusion testing for, 55

D
Dacarbazine, 216
Dactinomycin, 133t, 134t, 217
  extravasation of, 197t
Dactylitis, in sickle cell disease,
      22–23
Dancing eyes–dancing feet,
      in neuroblastoma, 188
Dapsone, prophylactic, 127
Daunomycin, 133t, 197t
Daunorubicin hydrochloride,
      217

DDAVP, 218–219
  in hemophilia-related hemor-
    rhage, 85, 87
  in von Willebrand disease,
    76–77, 78
Decadron, 133t
Deferoxamine mesylate, 61–62, 218
Delayed hemolytic transfusion
  reaction, 59
Desmopressin acetate, 218–219
  in hemophilia-related hemor-
    rhage, 85, 87
  in von Willebrand disease,
    76–77, 78
Dexamethasone, 219
  for vomiting, 134
Dimercaprol, 65, 220
Diphenhydramine, 220
  for vomiting, 135
  in nonhemolytic transfusion
    reaction, 58t
Diphtheria-pertussis-tetanus
  vaccine, 130t
Disseminated intravascular
  coagulation, 117
Doxorubicin hydrochloride,
  134t, 221
  extravasation of, 197t
Dronabinol, 221
Drugs. *See also specific generic*
  drugs.
  chemotherapy, 132t–133t
  extravasation of, 197–198, 197t
  generic names of, 199–201
  neutropenia with, 103
  pregnancy categories of, 203
  trade names of, 199–201
  vomiting with, 131–135, 134t

E

Edetate calcium disodium
  (EDTA), 222
  in treatment of lead toxicity, 65
Electrocardiography, in tumor
  lysis syndrome, 159

Elliptocytosis, hereditary, 4f, 11
Emesis, 131–135, 134t
EMLA, 224
Endocarditis, bacterial, prophylactic
  antibiotics for, 1287
Enoxaparin, 222–223
Ependymoma, 175
Epinephrine, in nonhemolytic
  transfusion reaction, 58t
Epistaxis
  in hemophilia, 89–91
  in von Willebrand disease, 77
Epoetin alfa, 8–9, 138, 223
Erythrocytapheresis, 50–51
Erythropoietin, 8–9, 138, 223
Esophagitis, 150
Etoposide, 133t, 134t, 224
Eutectic mixture of lidocaine and
  prilocaine, 224
Exchange transfusion, 50–51
  in hyperleukocytosis, 157
Extravasations, of chemotherapy,
  197–198, 197t

F

Factor V Leiden, mutation in,
  thromboembolism with, 94
Factor VIIa, recombinant, in
  hemophilia A, 89
Factor VIII
  deficiency of, 79–80
  in hemophilia-related hemor-
    rhage, 86t, 87t
  in von Willebrand disease, 78
  transfusion of, 53–54
Factor VIII coagulant, in
  von Willebrand disease, 76
Factor VIII inhibitors, in hemophilia A, 88–89
Factor IX
  deficiency of, 79–80
  in hemophilia-related
    hemorrhage, 86t, 87
Factor XI, deficiency of, 80
Factor XII, deficiency of, 81

Factor XIII, deficiency of, 80–81
Fanconi's anemia, 118
Ferritin, serum, 1
Ferrous gluconate, 225
Ferrous sulfate, 225
Fever, 145–152, 146f
  definition of, 145
  evaluation of, 145–147,
      146f
  in non-neutropenic patient,
      151–152
  in sickle cell disease,
      20–22, 21f
  management of, 147–148
  neutropenia with, 104–106,
      105f, 145–151, 146f
  persistent, 150–151
  transfusion-related, 57–58, 58t
Fibrinogen, in bleeding
    disorders, 70
Filgrastim, 135–136, 226
Fluconazole, 226–227
  prophylactic, 130
Fludarabine, 134t
Fluid therapy
  in hyperleukocytosis, 156
  in nonhemolytic transfusion
      reaction, 58t
  in tumor lysis syndrome, 158
Folate, 227
Folic acid, 227
Free erythrocyte protoporphyrin
    (FEP), 1, 2f
Fresh frozen plasma, 53–54
Fungal infection
  esophageal, 150
  prevention of, 130–131
  pulmonary, 150
  treatment of, 150–151

G

Gallstones, in sickle cell
    disease, 35
Gamma globulin, intravenous,
    in hemophilia A, 89

Ganciclovir, in viral infection, 149
Gastrointestinal bleeding, in
    sickle cell disease, 24
Gel electrophoresis, in
    von Willebrand disease, 76
Glucose-6-phosphate dehydroge-
    nase (G6PD) deficiency, 2t,
    4t, 7t, 13–14
Graft-versus-host disease,
    transfusion-related, 60
Granisetron, 131, 134, 228
Granulocyte transfusion,
    52–53
Granulocyte-colony-stimulating
    factor (G-CSF), 135–136,
    226
Granulocyte-macrophage
    colony-stimulating factor
    (GM-CSF), 137, 248
Growth factors, 135–138

H

Haemophilus influenzae type B
    vaccine, 130t
Hand-foot syndrome, in sickle cell
    disease, 22–23
Handwashing, 152
Headache, 119, 121t
  in sickle cell disease, 31
Hemangioma, 117–118
Hemarthroses, 83
Hematopoietic growth factors,
    135–138
Hematuria, 84
Hemoglobin
  in bleeding disorders, 68
  in sickle cell disease, 20
  normal, 3t
Hemoglobin E, 42, 43
Hemoglobin H, 40t, 41
Hemoglobin H–Constant Spring,
    40t, 41
Hemoglobin SC, 19
Hemoglobin SS, 19. *See also*
    Sickle cell disease.

Hemolytic anemia, 11–17
  evaluation of, 14–16, 15f
  in red cell enzyme defects,
    12–14
  in red cell membrane disorders,
    11–12
  treatment of, 16–17
Hemolytic transfusion reaction, 59
Hemophilia A, 79–80
  acute hemorrhage in, 83–91.
    See also Hemorrhage.
  epistaxis in, 89–91
  factor VIII inhibitors in, 88–89
Hemophilia B, 79–80
  acute hemorrhage in, 83–91.
    See also Hemorrhage.
  epistaxis in, 89–91
Hemophilia C, 80
Hemorrhage, 83–91
  dental, 84–85
  gastrointestinal, 84
  in neonatal alloimmune thrombo-
    cytopenia, 114
  in sickle cell disease, 32
  intracerebral, 32
  joint, 83
  mucosal, 84
  muscle, 83
  nasal, 89–91
  neurologic, 84
  retropharyngeal, 84
  subarachnoid, 32
  surgical, 84–85
  treatment of, 85–88, 86t
Hemostasis, 67
  disorders of, 67–72. See also
    Bleeding disorders.
Heparin sodium, 229
  in venous thrombosis, 97–100
Hepatitis A, 129t
Hepatitis B, 129t
Hepatitis B vaccine, 130t
Hereditary elliptocytosis, 11
Hereditary spherocytosis, 11–12
Herpes simplex virus infection,
  128–129, 149

High-molecular-weight kininogen
    deficiency, 81
Hodgkin's disease, 177–180
  clinical presentation of, 178
  diagnosis of, 178–179
  histology of, 177–178
  staging of, 179
  treatment of, 179–180
Horner's syndrome, in neuro-
    blastoma, 188
Hyaluronidase, 229–230
Hydrocortisone, 230
Hydromorphone hydrochloride, 231
Hydroxyurea, 134t, 231
Hyperbilirubinemia, in sickle cell
    disease, 35
Hyperkalemia, 157–159
Hyperleukocytosis, 120t, 122,
    155–157
Hyperphosphatemia, 157–159
Hyperuricemia, 157–159
Hyphema, in sickle cell disease, 35

I

Idarubicin, 134t, 232
Ifosfamide, 132t, 134t, 232
Iliopsoas muscle, bleeding into, 83
Immune globulin, 233
  intravenous
    in immune thrombocytopenic
      purpura, 112
    in neonatal alloimmune
      thrombocytopenia, 115
    in varicella zoster expo-
      sure, 128
  $Rh_0(D)$, 247
  varicella zoster, 128, 129t
Immune thrombocytopenic
    purpura, 107, 109–113
  chronic, 113
  evaluation of, 107, 109–112,
    110f, 111f
  treatment of, 112–113
Immune tolerance therapy,
    in hemophilia A, 89

Immunization, 129–130,
    129t, 130t
Infection
  Hodgkin's disease and, 177
  in non-neutropenic patient,
      151–152
  in sickle cell disease,
      20–22, 21f
  non-Hodgkin's lymphoma
      and, 180
  prevention of, 127–131, 129t,
      130t, 152
  transfusion-related, 60
  treatment of, 149
  with central venous catheter,
      141–142, 148–149
Influenza vaccine, 130t
Interferon alfa-2a, in Kasabach-
    Merritt syndrome, 118
International Normalized Ratio,
    in bleeding disorders, 69
Intracerebral hemorrhage, in sickle
    cell disease, 32
Intrathecal chemotherapy,
    191–192
Iron challenge, in anemia, 7–8
Iron complex, polysaccharide, 234
Iron deficiency anemia, 1–2,
    6–10
Iron dextran, 8, 233–234
Iron overload, 61
  chelation therapy for, 61–62
Iron therapy
  oral, 6–7
  parenteral, 8
Irradiation, for transfusion therapy,
    54–55

J
Joints, bleeding into, 83

K
Kasabach-Merritt syndrome,
    117–118

Ketorolac tromethamine, 235
Kidney, Wilms' tumor of, 183–185

L
Lead toxicity
  chelation therapy in, 64–65
  clinical effects of, 63
  prevention of, 63–64
Leucovorin calcium, 235–236
Leukapheresis, in hyperleuko-
    cytosis, 157
Leukemia
  acute, 161–168, 162t, 166t
  evaluation of, 122–124
  hyperleukocytosis in, 155–157
Leukocyte depletion, for transfusion
    therapy, 55
Leukocytosis, 120t, 122,
    155–157
Lidocaine, prilocaine mixture
    with, 224
Lomustine, 236
Lorazepam, for vomiting, 135
Low-molecular-weight heparin, in
    venous thrombosis, 97–100
Lumbar puncture
  in acute lymphoblastic leuke-
      mia, 163
  in brain tumor, 172
  in non-Hodgkin's
      lymphoma, 181
Lungs, infection of, 149, 150
  in sickle cell disease,
      26–29, 29f
Lymphadenopathy, 120–121,
    120t
Lymphoblastic leukemia, acute,
    161–166, 162t
Lymphoma
  Hodgkin's, 177–180
    clinical presentation of, 178
    diagnosis of, 178–179
    histology of, 177–178
    staging of, 179
    treatment of, 179–180

Lymphoma *(Continued)*
  non-Hodgkin's, 180–182
    clinical presentation of,
      180–181
    diagnosis of, 181
    treatment of, 181–182

M

Magnetic resonance imaging
  in brain tumor, 172
  in neuroblastoma, 189
May-Hegglin anomaly, 118
Mean corpuscular volume
    (MCV), 3, 3t
Measles, 129t
Measles-mumps-rubella vaccine,
    130t
Mechlorethamine, extravasation of,
    197t
Medulloblastoma, 173–174
Meningococcus vaccine, 130t
Meperidine hydrochloride, 237
6-Mercaptopurine, 132t,
    134t, 237
Mesna, 238
Methadone hydrochloride, 239
Methotrexate, 132t, 134t, 240
Methylprednisolone, 240–241
  in nonhemolytic transfusion
    reaction, 58t
Metoclopramide, 135, 241
Morphine sulfate, 242
  in nonhemolytic transfusion
    reaction, 58t
6-MP, 132t, 134t, 237
Muscle, bleeding into, 83
Mycostatin, oral, 130
Myelogenous leukemia, acute,
    166–168, 166t

N

Naloxone, 243
Necrotizing enterocolitis,
    of cecum, 155

Neonatal alloimmune neutro-
    penia, 103
Neonatal alloimmune thrombo-
    cytopenia, 113–115
Nephropathy, in sickle cell
    disease, 20
Neuroblastoma, 187–190
  clinical presentation of,
    187–188
  diagnosis of, 188–189
  staging of, 189
  treatment of, 189–190
Neutropenia, 101–106
  alloimmune, neonatal, 103
  benign, chronic, 101–102, 105f
  definition of, 101
  drug-induced, 103
  evaluation of, 104
  extrinsic causes of, 102–104
  fever and, 104–106, 105f,
    145–151, 146f
  in bacterial sepsis, 102–103
  in bone marrow replace-
    ment, 102
  in organomegaly, 103–104
  in viral infection, 102
  treatment of, 104–106, 105f
N-*myc,* in neuroblastoma,
    187, 190
Nosebleed
  in hemophilia, 89–91
  in von Willebrand disease, 77

O

Ommaya reservoir, tap and
    injection of, 193
Ondansetron, 131–135, 134t,
    243–244
Opsoclonus-myoclonus, in neuro-
    blastoma, 188
Oral hygiene, 127
Organomegaly, neutropenia with,
    103–104
Osteonecrosis, in sickle cell
    disease, 20

Oxygen therapy, in sickle cell disease, 27

P

Pain, in sickle cell disease, 22–26
Pancytopenia, 120t, 122
Parvovirus B19 infection, in sickle cell disease, 33
Patient-controlled analgesia, in sickle cell disease, 25–26
Pegaspargase, 244–245
Pentamidine, prophylactic, 127
Pentamidine isethionate, 245
Phytonadione, 254
Plasma, for transfusion therapy, 53–54
Plasminogen activator, tissue, 206
  in catheter-related thrombosis, 143
Platelet(s). See also Thrombocytopenia.
  in bleeding disorders, 69, 71t
  transfusion of, 51–52
    in neonatal alloimmune thrombocytopenia, 115
Pneumococcus vaccine, 130t
Pneumocystis carinii infection, 149
Pneumonia, in sickle cell disease, 26–29
Polio vaccine, 130, 130t
Porcine factor VIII concentrate, in hemophilia A, 89
Prednisone, 133t, 246
Prekallikrein deficiency, 81
Priapism, in sickle cell disease, 30
Prilocaine, lidocaine mixture with, 224
Procarbazine hydrochloride, 132t, 246–247
Promethazine, for vomiting, 135
Protein C deficiency, thromboembolism with, 94
Protein S deficiency, thromboembolism with, 94

Prothrombin, mutation in, thromboembolism with, 94
Prothrombin time, in bleeding disorders, 69, 71t
Pulmonary embolism, in sickle cell disease, 27
Pulmonary hypertension, in sickle cell disease, 20
Pyruvate kinase deficiency, 13

R

Radiation therapy
  in brain tumor, 173
  vomiting with, 131–135, 134t
Red cell distribution index (RDW), 1, 2f
Retinoic acid, in acute myelogenous leukemia, 168
Retinopathy, in sickle cell disease, 20, 34–35
Retrosternal pain, 150
Rh$_0$(D) immune globulin, 113, 247
Ristocetin cofactor, in von Willebrand disease, 76

S

Sargramostim (GM-CSF), 137, 248
Sepsis
  neutropenia in, 102–103
  with central venous catheter, 142
Serotonin antagonists, for emesis prevention, 131–135, 134t
Sickle cell disease, 19–38
  abdominal pain in, 23
  acute chest syndrome in, 26–29, 29f
  anemia in, 32–33
  aplastic crisis in, 33
  avascular necrosis in, 33–34
  dactylitis in, 22–23
  fever in, 20–22, 21f
  gallstones in, 35
  gastrointestinal bleeding in, 24

Sickle cell disease (Continued)
  hyperbilirubinemia in, 35
  hyphema in, 35
  infection, 20–22, 21f
  musculoskeletal pain in, 23
  pain in, 22–26
  patient-controlled analgesia in,
    25–26
  preoperative care in, 35–36
  priapism in, 30
  retinopathy in, 34–35
  splenic sequestration in, 32–33
  stroke in, 30–32
  transfusion therapy in, 48–49
  vaso-occlusive episodes in,
    22–26
Spherocytosis, hereditary, 11–12
Spine, tumors of, 171–172
Spirometry, in sickle cell
    disease, 26
Splenectomy
  in hereditary spherocytosis, 12
  in pyruvate kinase deficiency, 13
  in sickle cell disease, 32–33
Splenic sequestration, in sickle cell
    disease, 32–33
Straddle injury, 84
Stroke, in sickle cell disease,
    30–32
Subarachnoid hemorrhage,
    in sickle cell disease, 32
Succimer, 64–65, 248
Sulfamethoxazole-trimethoprim,
    127, 149, 249
Superior vena cava syndrome,
    153–154
Surgery
  in brain tumor, 173
  in neuroblastoma, 190
  in sickle cell disease, 35–36

T

Testes, in acute lymphoblastic
    leukemia, 162
6-TG, 132t, 134t, 250

à-Thalassemia, 19, 39–42, 40t
  silent carrier in, 39–40, 40t
á-Thalassemia, 40t, 42–45
  screening for, 45
Thalassemia intermedia,
    43–44
à-Thalassemia major, 40t, 42
á-Thalassemia major, 44–45
à-Thalassemia trait, 40t, 41
á-Thalassemia trait, 42–43
Thioguanine, 250
6-Thioguanine, 132t, 134t, 250
Thiotepa, 134t, 250
Thrombin, topical, 251
Thrombin time, in bleeding
    disorders, 70
Thrombocytopenia
  alloimmune, neonatal,
    113–115
  amegakaryocytic, congenital, 118
  drug-induced, 115
  immune-mediated, 107–116,
    108t–109t, 109f, 110f,
    111f
    differential diagnosis of,
      108t–109t
    evaluation of, 109f, 110f,
      111f
  in sick newborn, 117
  non–immune-mediated,
    117–118
  platelet transfusion in, 51–52
Thrombocytopenia–absent radii
    syndrome, 118
Thrombocytopenic purpura
  idiopathic, chronic, 113
  immune, 107, 109–113
    evaluation of, 107, 109–112,
      110f, 111f
    treatment of, 112–113
Thrombosis, venous, 93–100
  anticoagulation therapy for, 95,
    97–100
  low-molecular-weight heparin in,
    97–100
  patient history in, 95

Thrombosis, venous *(Continued)*
  physical examination in,
    95, 96f
  prothrombotic disorders and,
    94–95, 94t
  risk factors for, 93–94
  standard heparin in, 97
  with central venous catheter,
    141, 142–143
Tissue plasminogen activator,
    206
  in catheter-related thrombo-
    sis, 143
Tranexamic acid, 251
  in hemophilia-related
    hemorrhage, 87–88
  in von Willebrand disease, 77
Transcranial Doppler examination,
    in sickle cell disease, 31
Transferrin saturation, 1
Transfusion reactions, 57–60
  allergic, 57
  alloimmunization, 59
  bacteria-related, 60
  graft-versus-host, 60
  hemolytic, 59
  nonhemolytic, febrile,
    57–58, 58t
Transfusion therapy, 47–55
  antithrombin III for, 54
  cytomegalovirus testing
    for, 55
  granulocytes for, 52–53
  in anemia, 9–10
  in cancer patient, 49–50
  in neonatal alloimmune
    thrombocytopenia, 115
  in sickle cell disease, 29,
    36–37, 48–49
  irradiation for, 54–55
  leukocyte depletion for, 55
  plasma for, 53–54
  platelets for, 51–52
  red blood cells for, 47–51
    dosage of, 50–51
    indications for, 48

Transient ischemic attack, in sickle
    cell disease, 31–32
Trimethoprim-sulfamethoxazole, 249
  in *Pneumocystis carinii* infec-
    tion, 149
  prophylactic, 127
Tuberculosis, 129t
Tumor lysis syndrome, 157–159
Typhlitis, 155

U

Urate oxidase, 252
  in hyperleukocytosis, 156
  in tumor lysis syndrome, 158
Urokinase, 252
  in catheter-related thrombo-
    sis, 143

V

Vaccines, 129–130, 129t,
    130t
Varicella vaccine, 130t
Varicella zoster immune globulin,
    128, 129t
Varicella zoster virus infection,
    128, 129t, 149
Vaso-occlusive episodes, in sickle
    cell disease, 22–26
Venous
  thrombosis, 93–100. *See also*
    Thrombosis, venous.
Vinblastine sulfate, 133t,
    134t, 253
  extravasation of, 197t
Vincristine sulfate, 133t, 134t,
    253–254
  extravasation of, 197t
Vindesine, extravasation of, 197t
Viral infection
  in hereditary spherocytosis, 12
  neutropenia with, 102
  prevention of, 128–130,
    129t
  treatment of, 149

Vitamin K$_1$, 254
Vomiting, 131–135, 134t
Von Willebrand disease, 75–81
    acquired, 78
    clinical presentation of, 75–76
    diagnosis of, 76
    treatment of, 76–78
Von Willebrand factor antigen, 76
VP-16, 133t, 134t, 224

W

Warfarin sodium, 255
Wilms' tumor, 183–185
    clinical presentation of, 183
    diagnosis of, 183–184
    genetics of, 183
    staging of, 184–185
    treatment of, 185
Wiskott-Aldrich syndrome, 118

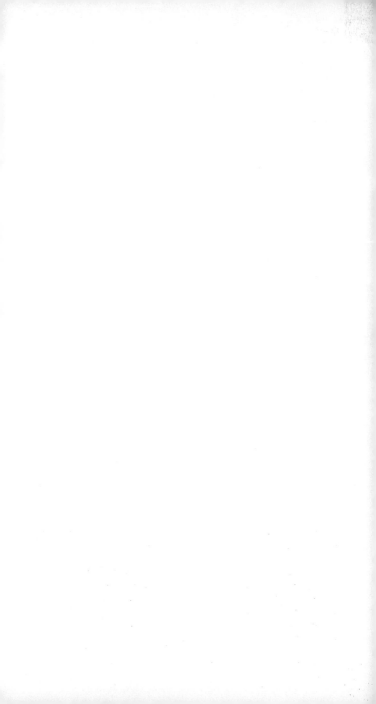